The Complete DASH Diet Guide

Lose Weight, Lower Blood Pressure and Prevent Diabetes

Melanie Fletcher

Contents

Introduction

High blood pressure is a big problem being faced by the world today. Did you know that over a billion people are affected by high blood pressure? This number does not seem to be going down either. It's becoming a serious concern that we're all faced with on a daily basis. High blood pressure leads to a number of dangerous conditions like heart disease, kidney failure, and stroke.

Our diet plays a huge role in this epidemic, so that means we need to develop better eating habits if we are going to keep from becoming part of this statistic. That's where the DASH diet enters the picture. This dieting plan was developed by scientists and doctors with one specific goal in mind—to combat high blood pressure.

This book is going to dive deep into the DASH diet to help you counter the dangerous lifestyle that encompasses Western dieting.

Why is DASH Dieting so Healthy?

First and foremost, it was designed by the National Heart, Lung, and Blood Institute (NHLBI) to lower blood pressure in patients. Therefore, it's considered to be one of the healthiest eating plans for lowering blood pressure. All you have to do in order to follow through with this diet is reduce your intake of unhealthy fats, refined sugar, and sodium. There are not that many restrictions.

The food options are quite vast, putting an emphasis on whole foods like vegetables and fruit, fat-free dairy products, lean meats, and whole grains. It also eliminates processed foods, simple sugars, and packaged snacks. It's also encouraged that you limit red meats.

Processed foods do not taste that great anyway. You just think they do now because your palate is out of balance. Once you clean up your eating habits, you'll wonder why you ever ate those foods in the first place!

The DASH diet also limits sodium intake, which can give you an edge over hypertension and also help lose weight. This is a great choice for individuals who might have a family history of heart disease or those at risk of type-2 diabetes.

On average, the DASH dieting plan will include the following foods on a daily basis:

- ➢ 8 servings of whole grains
- ➢ 6 servings of meat
- ➢ 5 servings of vegetables
- ➢ 4 servings of fruit
- ➢ 2-3 servings of fat-free dairy products

Introduction

- 2 servings of oils

Some of the daily goals will include:

- Fat should never be more than 27% of your calorie intake, with saturated fat making up no more than 6% of that.

- Protein should be 18% of your calorie intake.

- Carbohydrates should be 55% of your total calorie intake

- Never consume more than 150 mg of cholesterol

- Consume at least 30 grams of fiber

As you can see, this is a lifestyle choice. It doesn't rely on giving up one area of nutrition to boost another. It's not based on some fad with no scientific evidence to support it. It simply involves making better food choices and paying attention to what you're putting into your body.

Are you ready to get started?

Part 1

DASH Diet

Basics

Chapter 1

What Exactly is the DASH Diet?

DASH is an acronym that stands for "Dietary Approaches to Stop Hypertension."

It's a dieting approach that is recommended to individuals who are looking to reduce their blood pressure. DASH dieting puts your focus on fruits, vegetables, whole grains, and lean meats.

Once high blood pressure started becoming such a huge problem, experts searched for answers. It wasn't that difficult to find the reason for the sudden spike in numbers. We have become too reliant on fast food and processed food—both of which are detrimental to our health. As a result, we have moved away from whole foods in favor of convenience. The DASH diet is designed to help us move back to those healthier whole foods.

DASH dieting puts our focus back onto fruits and vegetables while eliminating those nasty processed foods from our lifestyle. It also puts a focus on healthier proteins like fish, poultry, and beans.

One of the biggest contributors to low blood pressure is the fact that this diet naturally reduces the amount of sodium being put into your body. Processed foods are loaded with sodium, so the simple step of avoiding them will make a huge difference.

There are actually two different forms of the DASH diet that people can choose to follow depending on how out of balance their blood pressure is.

The Standard DASH Diet encourages you to limit yourself to no more than 2,300 mg of sodium per day.

The Lower-Sodium DASH Diet encourages you to limit yourself to no more than 1,500 mg of sodium per day.

We will look at these in more detail later in this chapter. But right now, I want you to understand that the DASH diet focuses on whole foods and restricts sodium. This takes a little bit of getting used to since your taste buds are accustomed to getting bombarded with salty foods on a daily basis. However, it only takes a week or two for you to adapt to the lessened amount of salt.

So now let's look at the benefits of DASH dieting. Blood pressure is the measurement used to show how much force is put on organs and blood vessels as your blood pumps through them. There are two different numbers used:

Systolic Pressure: This is the pressure put on blood vessels every time your heart beats.

Diastolic Pressure: This is the pressure put on your blood vessels between heart beats.

Normal blood pressure has a systolic pressure of 120 and a diastolic pressure of 80. It's usually written as 120/80. Individuals whose blood pressure measures at 140/90 or above are considered to have high blood pressure.

What is interesting is that the DASH diet has been shown to lower blood pressure for both healthy people and those whose blood pressure is already high. This has also been achieved in people who did not lose weight as a result of the diet, although most people who follow the DASH diet will experience weight loss.

There is a direct correlation between people who consume a lower amount of sodium and those who experience the highest reduction in blood pressure. My point here is that the DASH diet is one of the most effective ways to lower blood pressure. That's always going to be your primary goal.

Can the DASH Diet Lead to Weight Loss?

So we know that the DASH diet was designed with blood pressure in mind, but where does it stand on weight loss? For starters, if you have been diagnosed with high blood pressure then chances are that you have been told that you need to lose weight. That's because weight has a direct impact on blood pressure. When we gain weight, our blood pressure rises, and when we lose weight, it goes down.

My point is that weight loss can be a side-effect of DASH dieting, but you should always remember that it's not what the dieting plan was designed to do. With that in mind, another important part of lowering your blood pressure is to reduce your calorie intake. The DASH diet is designed to do that because it promotes whole foods over their processed counterparts. A reduction in calorie intake will give you a much greater chance of losing weight. As you move forward with this new lifestyle, you might have to consciously start making adjustments that ensure you remain at a calorie deficit.

If you are looking to lose weight, then eating the foods that are listed on the DASH Diet is going to make it much easy to restrict your calorie intake. Eventually, you will need to start tracking your calories in order to ensure that you are at a calorie deficit.

So in short, the DASH Diet can be an amazing tool to help you lose weight, but you will still have to make sure that you remain at a calorie deficit.

Potential Health Benefits of the DASH Diet

By this point, we know that the DASH Diet was designed to lower blood pressure, so we already know that benefit. Let's look at some of the other potential benefits.

It can decrease your risk of cancer. There are some experts who believe that this diet can help lower the risk of certain cancers. The main focus of studies has been on breast cancer and colorectal cancer. In these cases, there is evidence that seems to support a decrease in the risk of cancer.

It lowers the risk of metabolic syndrome. This dieting plan can potentially reduce your chances of developing metabolic syndrome.

It reduces your chances of developing diabetes. People who follow the DASH diet have been shown to have a lower risk of developing type-2 diabetes. The reason is because this diet encourages us to eat more whole foods. Diets rich in whole foods, while reducing our intake of processed foods and refined sugars, have been proven to lower the risk of diabetes.

It lowers the risk of heart disease. Since the DASH Diet is designed to lower blood pressure, it's also going to reduce your chances of developing heart disease and even strokes.

DASH Dieting is one of the easiest diets to follow. Since the only requirements are that you eat more whole foods and avoid processed choices, you will find that you have a lot of choices when it comes to meal selection. This makes it one of the easiest diets to follow through with for the long-term.

It lowers cholesterol levels. One of the major causes of high blood pressure is the consumption of too much bad cholesterol. Whole foods are lower in bad cholesterol, so they are naturally going to lower your cholesterol levels.

DASH Dieting can potentially lead to weight loss. This is the goal that many of us have, so it's important to note that this diet can help you lose weight since it focuses on foods that are high in fiber, protein, and other essential nutrients.

These benefits are the result of eating a diet that is higher in fruits and vegetables. Following a healthier lifestyle will reduce your risks of certain diseases.

Does it Work for Everyone?
One of the key factors with any dieting plan is consistency. Following a healthy diet that you can actually stick with is essential. There is no dieting plan in the world that will work for everyone since all of us are unique. With that in mind, it was designed to reduce blood pressure, and it can accomplish that goal. But that will do you little good if you can't follow through with it.

The greatest reduction in blood pressure is experienced by those who follow the low sodium version which is no surprise since reduction in salt intake has been shown to significantly reduce blood pressure.

My point here is that lowering your intake of salt while swapping over to whole foods is a much healthier lifestyle, but you have to make sure that any dieting plan is suited for your personal taste.

Chapter 2
Minerals and Their Role

Minerals are an essential part of your health, so when following through with a new diet, it's important that you make sure you are getting all of the essentials. Your body must have these essential minerals in order to grow and develop.

There are two types of minerals–macrominerals and trace minerals. Macrominerals are required in rather large quantities. Macrominerals include:

 ➢ Calcium
 ➢ Phosphorus
 ➢ Magnesium
 ➢ Sodium
 ➢ Potassium
 ➢ Sulfur
 ➢ Chloride

Our bodies also need trace minerals, but they are only needed in very small amounts. Trace minerals include:

 ➢ Iron
 ➢ Zinc
 ➢ Manganese
 ➢ Copper

- ➢ Iodine
- ➢ Fluoride
- ➢ Cobalt
- ➢ Selenium

Let's take a closer look at some of these important nutrients to see what role they play.

Calcium, Phosphorus, and Magnesium

Calcium is the most abundant mineral in our body. It is used in bones and teeth while also playing a vital role in muscle contraction. We must have calcium in order to survive.

Main Sources of Calcium

- ➢ Leafy green vegetables
- ➢ Dairy products

Phosphorus is used to repair our cells and generate DNA. Needless to say, both of those roles are extremely important to our survival.

Main Sources of Phosphorus

- ➢ Nuts
- ➢ Poultry
- ➢ Meat
- ➢ Eggs
- ➢ Fish
- ➢ Legumes

Finally, magnesium is used to fuel our energy production and regulates our calcium levels. Lacking this mineral will cause us to feel sluggish.

Main Sources of Magnesium

- ➤ Whole grains
- ➤ Black walnuts
- ➤ Almonds
- ➤ Cashews
- ➤ Green leafy vegetables

Sodium, Potassium, and Chloride

We must have sodium in order to survive since it plays a vital role in regulating our blood pressure and volume. The problem is that too much sodium can have a negative impact. DASH dieters should be cautious about how much sodium they consume.

Main Sources of Sodium

- ➤ Table salt
- ➤ Sodium chloride
- ➤ Celery
- ➤ Milk
- ➤ Beets

Potassium helps conduct electricity in our body, otherwise known as an electrolyte. It supports a healthy heart and muscular functions throughout the body.

Main Sources of Potassium

> ➤ Salmon
> ➤ Fish
> ➤ Legumes
> ➤ Dairy
> ➤ Bananas
> ➤ Most vegetables

Chloride will help your body maintain a balance of fluids.

Main Sources of Chloride

> ➤ Seaweed
> ➤ Lettuce
> ➤ Olives
> ➤ Rye
> ➤ Tomatoes

Iron, Zinc, Manganese, and Copper

Iron is an essential part of our red blood cells, which in turn provide oxygen to tissues in the body.

Main Sources of Iron

> ➤ Eggs

➢ Beans
➢ Leafy green vegetables
➢ Dried fruits

Zinc promotes a healthy immune system and also helps contribute to cellular growth.

Main Sources of Zinc

➢ Nuts
➢ Legumes
➢ Lean beef
➢ Lean pork

Manganese is used by the body to create connective tissues, hormones, and helps our bones repair.

Main Sources of Manganese

➢ Whole grains
➢ Nuts
➢ Seeds
➢ Pineapple

Copper promotes the health of your nerves and immune system.

Main Sources of Copper

➢ Seafood
➢ Organ meats

- ➤ Black pepper
- ➤ Legumes
- ➤ Fruits
- ➤ Vegetables

Iodine, Fluoride, and Selenium

Iodine assists in the creation of thyroid hormones, which are an essential part of growth. This is an important nutrient.

Main Sources of Iodine

- ➤ Lima Beans
- ➤ Sesame seeds
- ➤ Spinach
- ➤ Swiss chard
- ➤ Turnip greens
- ➤ Summer squash

Fluoride helps keep your teeth healthy and plays an important role in maintaining bone structure. Most drinking water contains fluoride.

Main Sources of Fluoride

- ➤ Seafood
- ➤ Gelatin
- ➤ Tea

Selenium is essential to healthy thyroid function and will also help your immune system function better.

Main Sources of Selenium

- ➢ Brewer's yeast
- ➢ Butter
- ➢ Garlic
- ➢ Sunflower seeds
- ➢ Brazil nuts
- ➢ Wheat germ

Chapter 3
A Quick Word About Alcohol

Now we're going to discuss a topic that's left out in a lot of other dieting books. It's an issue that many people ask me about, so I feel compelled to include an entire chapter. Does being on the DASH diet mean that you have to completely give up drinking?

First of all, it's fairly obvious that drinking too much is not healthy. It can wreak havoc on all of our health-related goals. That's not exactly groundbreaking news. But does having that one night cap really become a catalyst that will unravel everything that you have worked so hard to achieve?

The short answer is no. One drink is not going to sink your fitness goals. However, drinking regularly is going tomake your goals so much more difficult to achieve. So if you want to grab an occasional drink without losing your way, then keep reading. After all, I am pretty adamant in my stance when it comes to 90% compliance. Being too strict will cause your new lifestyle to become stale. If it's stale, you will eventually fall off the wagon.

How Alcohol Can Stall Your Health Goals
Alcohol can actually stall your health-related goals in more ways than you might imagine. First of all, it stimulates your

appetite and makes you crave unhealthy foods. You'll be reaching for those starchy, sauce covered foods like fries and hot wings! Your body does not register the calories from alcoholic beverages, so you will not eat less to compensate. You'll actually end up eating more.

We consider alcohol empty calories since you get no nutritional value from it. Wasted calories make it much more difficult to achieve your goals.

Furthermore, alcohol will also impair your body's ability to digest food. So you are not going to get all of the valuable nutrients from the foods you eat while consuming alcohol.

Companies are also not required to label the nutritional information for alcoholic beverages, so that's another hurdle that you have to overcome. It's essential that you are able to track what you are putting into your body, so you will have to research the nutritional information about any alcohol you consume. Some breweries do include nutritional information on their products, so you can also choose to buy these too.

I am going to walk you through several do's and don'ts of alcohol.

<u>DO</u> limit yourself to no more than two drinks.

Alcohol in moderation can be a part of a healthy lifestyle. The problem is that we all tend to have a different definition for the term "in moderation." For the purpose of DASH dieting, you should not have more than two drinks on any given day. You should also try to limit alcohol consumption to no more than three days a week.

<u>DO</u> understand what a "drink" really is.

A "drink" is seen as completely different sizes depending on who you're talking to. As a rule of thumb, here are some drink sizes that you should follow:

➢ 5-ounce glass of wine
➢ 1.5-ounce shot if liquor
➢ 12-ounce bottle of beer

Remember, you should not consume more than two drinks in a day.

<u>DON'T</u> have mixed drinks.

Cocktails are loaded with sugar and add even more empty calories to your diet. Plus, sugary drinks are one of the biggest things that we need to avoid on the DASH diet. Additionally, they are usually served in large sizes. Just a 9-ounce piña colada is loaded with a whopping 490 calories! That's 25% of your daily calories in one drink.

<u>DO</u> drink a lot of water.

Alcohol dehydrates your body, so when you drink it, you will have to drink even more water to compensate. Try drinking a full glass of water before your first drink or order your drinks with lots of ice. Staying hydrated is one of the most important parts of living a healthier lifestyle.

DON'T believe everything you read about alcohol.

Yes, there are a lot of studies out there that link alcohol to benefits like a lower risk of heart disease and even some studies that show it can help stave off diabetes. However, that does not mean that these benefits outweigh the risks. Furthermore, these benefits are all based on just having one drink per day. You'll be hard-pressed to find an expert who would recommend you to start drinking if you currently don't drink.

DO sip and savor your drink.

You should develop a healthy mindset about drinking. Don't drink to help deal with stress or to improve your life. You should drink for the enjoyment of having a delicious beverage. There are healthier ways to deal with stress. When you start savoring your drink, you will develop a healthier mindset about it.

DON'T use alcohol as a way to sleep better.

So many people do this, and it actually has the opposite effect. Sure, alcohol is a sedative and will help you nod off, but it will disrupt your sleep cycle. It reduces the amount of time you stay in REM sleep, which is why you feel groggy waking up after drinking the previous night.

Chapter 4
Foods to Avoid

One of the biggest concerns with any dieting plan is to learn what foods you can eat and what foods you have to avoid. While the DASH diet is not as restrictive as most diets, you still need to avoid certain foods. In short, you will be replacing all of those processed foods with whole foods. Eat more fruits and vegetables while avoiding foods high in sodium. Here are a few examples of changes that you'll be making to your diet.

➢ Eat a salad with some added protein instead of grabbing a burger and fries.
➢ Choose low-fat Greek yogurt rather than sweetened yogurt.
➢ Eat whole oatmeal rather than the sweetened processed oatmeal packs.
➢ Avoid the vending machine, and grab a piece of fruit or raw veggie sticks as a snack.
➢ Replace processed grains with whole grains like brown rice.
➢ Replace all of those greasy burgers with lean proteins like chicken and fish.

What Should Be Avoided?

There are several foods that you should avoid when following the DASH diet. Again, you are avoiding foods that are high in sugar, sodium, and processed foods. Here are some examples:

➢ Candy
➢ Cookies
➢ Chips
➢ Salted nuts
➢ Sodas
➢ Sugary beverages including fruit juice
➢ Pastries
➢ Meat dishes
➢ Prepackaged pasta dishes (example: Hamburger Helper)
➢ Prepackaged rice dishes
➢ Pizza
➢ Soups
➢ Cheese
➢ Cured meats
➢ White bread
➢ Sandwiches
➢ Gravy
➢ Canned soups

You can use a salt substitute that is created from potassium. It not only works wonderfully, but the added potassium will actually help regulate your blood pressure. Individuals who are on blood pressure medications should be sure to ask their doctors about consuming additional potassium, though, since you can actually overdose on this nutrient.

A Word About Red Meat

While you can enjoy the occasional serving of red meat, you should always choose grass-fed options over their traditional grain-fed counterparts. Grass-fed beef is high in omega-3s and is actually similar to fish in its nutritional makeup. Traditional grain-fed red meat should be avoided since it is loaded with saturated fat, a big contributor to heart disease.

If you don't think that you can completely remove red meat from your diet, just try to limit your consumption to no more than two to three servings per week. I do not believe in completely restricting foods on any dieting plan. Your goal should always be 90% compliance.

A Few Changes Can Make a World of Difference

The DASH diet dictates a specific number of servings from certain food groups each day. While you can certainly follow it as strictly as you want, those who are more flexible tend to find the most success. Here are a few small changes that you can make to your diet that will get you on the right path.

Half of Your Plate Should be Vegetables and/or Fruit
You should be eating five servings vegetables and five servings of fruits every day. In order to achieve this goal, you should start filling up half of your plate with vegetables and fruit with every meal. Following this simple rule will make a world of difference.

Start your day with a side of fruit, and try adding an extra serving of veggies with your breakfast. For example, try making an avocado spread to put onto your toast.

At lunch, add double the usual amount of vegetables to your plate. Also try scaling up the amount of vegetables you put in dishes like stir fry and stews. That will get you a few extra servings from standard meals.

Adding a salad as a snack between meals is also another great way to add more vegetables to your everyday routine.

The point here is to become proactive in adding more vegetables and fruits to your standard routine. One of the most efficient ways to successfully follow through with any new dieting plan is to find ways to incorporate it into your daily routine. The fewer changes you make, the more likely you are to achieve long-term success.

Get in a Few Servings of Low-Fat Dairy Every Day
Another staple of the DASH diet are low-fat dairy products. These foods are loaded with essential nutrients and vitamins.

In fact, many experts believe that the calcium and potassium found in dairy products can help manage blood pressure.

Low-fat yogurt is an amazing breakfast option. Just add in some fruit for flavor, and you're good to go! You can also add milk to your homemade smoothies or grab some cheese to enjoy as an afternoon snack.

If you are lactose intolerant, then you can replace dairy with a non-dairy alternative like almond milk.

Replace Starchy Snacks with Whole Food

DASH dieting requires that you avoid all of those vending machine snacks like chips, cookies, and even those processed nuts. You should replace those snacks with whole foods.

- ➢ Instead of grabbing a pack of crackers, try snacking on a palm full of nuts.
- ➢ Rather than getting a candy bar, try eating an apple.
- ➢ Enjoy an afternoon salad rather than a bag of chips.

You need to focus on whole foods. It will keep your calorie count down and helps you budget your foods correctly. Here are a few snack choices that are DASH diet friendly:

- ➢ Celery sticks with a small amount of nut butter
- ➢ Whole grain crackers topped with cheese
- ➢ Low-fat yogurt with added fruit
- ➢ Palm full of nuts

➤ Veggie sticks with hummus

Replace Red Meat with Healthier Meats

You should replace most red meat with beans, fish, or poultry. DASH dieters should aim for approximately six ounces of lean protein every day. We see plenty of poultry in the Western diet, but most people skip the beans and fish. Furthermore, poultry should be eaten with the skin removed since it contains so much saturated fat.

You can make soups or add protein to salads. I recommend that you go meatless one or two days a week, and replace meats with beans on those days.

Chapter 5

Nutrients and Their Role in Our Diet

There are literally hundreds of thousands of different foods around the world, and most of them are based on the three essential nutrients–carbs, fats, and protein. Those three essential building blocks are called macronutrients by scientists. For the purposes of dieting, we refer to them as macros. Each macronutrient has a specific number of calories that you will get from them. You will eat a specific breakdown of carbs, fats, and protein.

These macros are important to living a healthier life. The best way to describe this is to look at your body like a car. Macros are the fuel for your body. You must give it the right amount in order to survive. However, if you give it the best possible blend, then your body will thrive. We are all biologically designed to get a specific ratio of these macronutrients.

You have probably heard of the ketogenic diet where people closely monitor their macros so that they are eating more fat. Macros are also an important part of the DASH diet because you want to make sure you are getting the right amount of nutrients. Let's take a closer look at macronutrients and their effect on our body.

Everyone Has Different Needs

There are a lot of different factors that affect our required macros. This can include blood markers, genetics, level of activity, medical conditions, and even your metrics.

When you are eating the right macros, you will start to feel much better. You can also see the benefits through your health markers like cholesterol, triglycerides, and fasting blood glucose. If these numbers are high, then it's probably because you are not following the right macros. The DASH Diet will help make it easier to get in the right combination since you're focusing on whole foods. It's still important to keep track though.

Eating the wrong combination of foods will actually make you feel worse. You'll struggle in the afternoon because your energy will suddenly dwindle. These energy crashes are common symptoms associated with the standard Western diet. They are brought on from eating too many carbs and not getting enough fats and protein.

Not Everyone Can Benefit from a High Fat Diet

This is a fact that all of those ketogenic diet backers seem to forget. Some people are not going to benefit from a high-fat diet because it will cause their cholesterol to become elevated. That's where DASH dieting comes into play. It's amazing how two people can respond so differently to the same nutrient.

It's usually related to genetics and lifestyle. Genes can cause our bodies to handle fat in completely different ways. For instance, the APO gene can come in different variations, some of which are associated with higher than normal triglyceride levels.

Genetics are complex, though, so having that variant doesn't necessarily mean you will have high triglycerides. Individual genetics don't always have an impact on the way you handle fat. It's a very complicated topic that is based on your unique makeup.

In fact, some individuals have no problem consuming a high-carb diet, so they can be more flexible with their carb intake. That's why some people have bad results from the ketogenic diet. It's also why some people can seemingly eat a lot of junk food and never gain weight.

One thing that impacts everyone is activity. The more active you are, the healthier your body will be.

Some People Must Have More Protein

We're not just talking about bodybuilders here either. People who are in their 60s and have elevated blood pressure will benefit from added proteins. Protein is also a great way to manage your blood sugar levels. People trying to lose weight can also benefit from eating more protein because it helps build lean muscle mass, which in turn boosts your metabolism.

Protein is clearly beneficial, but the reasoning behind it is not always clear. Let me try to explain. One theory behind the lowered blood sugar levels is that animal proteins are believed to have higher levels of arginine, which is a natural deterrent of high blood pressure.

Finally, eating more proteins will also cause you to eat fewer calories because they sustain you for longer than carbs.

Our Body Changes Over Time

I'm sure you have all heard that metabolism slows down as we get older. This is not necessarily accurate. What really happens is that our body burns calories more slowly as we get older. There is a distinct difference. Again, this is not going to be true for everyone. More active people tend to continue burning calories efficiently as they get older.

For example, a person who can gorge themselves on fast food in their 20s without gaining weight will find that they will eventually start packing away those calories as they get older. They rapidly gain weight, and their cholesterol goes through the roof! The reason is because their body eventually stops processing those calories at a rapid pace.

Macros Help You Focus Your Efforts

When you understand how macros work, you can break them down in a way that will help you achieve your goals. It helps you focus on planning rather than guessing. For instance, if you know that your body processes a high-carb diet better than a high-fat diet, then you can adjust your foods in a way that you're consuming more carbs.

Cholesterol

Cholesterol is a substance this flows through our blood. It's almost waxy in nature. The body uses it in order to create cells and hormones. Our liver creates all of the required cholesterol needed from fats that are consumed in our diet.

The problem is that it does not dissolve in the blood. Rather, it bonds with lipoproteins which will transport it between cells. These carriers are comprised of fat on the inside and protein on the outside. This is important to understand because cholesterol can build up in our arteries and clog them, leading to severe issues like a heart attack or stroke.

Good Cholesterol Versus Bad Cholesterol

There are two very distinct types of cholesterol that are treated in two entirely different ways. The bad cholesterol is carried by low-density lipoproteins (LDL) which can accumulate in arteries and lead to severe heart conditions. The other type of cholesterol is carried by high-density lipoproteins (HDL) from other areas of the body and back to the liver, which will then process the cholesterol out of the body. It's important that you have a healthy level of both types of cholesterol, but the good will essentially help remove excess bad cholesterol.

If your cholesterol levels become too high then it will start to deposit in your arteries. These fatty, waxy deposits will build up on the walls of your blood vessels and make it harder for blood to flow through, leading to higher blood pressure. This is known as atherosclerosis.

Narrow vessels can only transport a limited amount of oxygen, which can lead to a heart attack or a stroke.

Healthy Levels of Cholesterol
Cholesterol is measured in milligrams per tenth-liter (mg/dl). This measurement should always be below 200 mg/dl. Lower numbers tend to lower your risk factors for heart disease.

> ➢ Bad cholesterol (LDL) should be less than 160 mg/dl.
> ➢ Good cholesterol (HDL) should measure at least 35 mg/dl.

Higher levels of good cholesterol will give you better protection against heart disease because it helps remove the bad.

What's amazing is that over 30% of Americans have high levels of LDL cholesterol. This is due to the overconsumption of processed foods and sugars. Of that 30%, only half of them are even aware that they have a problem. Even then, they don't take steps to correct it until they suffer severe side effects (like a mild heart attack or stroke).

Individuals who have high cholesterol have twice the risk for heart disease as those who maintain healthy levels. There are certain drugs that can treat high cholesterol, but the only long-term solution is to make sure you are eating the right foods. That is one of the main goals behind the DASH diet.

It's highly recommended that everyone have their cholesterol checked every five years. Testing is the only way you know for sure where you stand.

What Are the Risk Factors?
While your diet is certainly one of the most prominent risk factors that can lead to the development of high cholesterol, there are other factors that many people don't consider. One is age. As we get older, our risk for developing high cholesterol increases. This is especially true for women who go through menopause.

Genetics also play a role since they determine how much cholesterol your liver creates. Watch out for a family history of high blood pressure or heart disease because that could mean that you're more susceptible to high cholesterol.

Genetics and age are two factors that you can't control, but you can reduce your risk in other areas. Physical activity will reduce your levels of cholesterol. You can also reduce the amount of saturated fat in your diet. If you smoke, then you should quit immediately because it will damage your blood vessels.

Preventing High Cholesterol in Two Easy Steps

The first step to preventing high cholesterol is to eat a healthy diet. That's what the DASH diet is designed to do. You'll want to reduce your consumption of processed foods, which tend to be loaded in saturated fats. Instead, eat whole foods that are loaded with healthy fats. Switch over to lean, skinless meats for starters. Eat more whole vegetables and fruits. Load up on whole grains and snack on nuts. DASH dieting is not as restrictive as most diets, so you will have a lot of different foods to choose from.

The next step is to lose weight and exercise. Exercise is optional, and I'm going to actually show you how to make every day choices that make you more active. But if your cholesterol is dangerously high, then you might need to devote time to exercising.

Losing weight will also help keep your cholesterol levels under control. So if you are obese, then you should create a few weight loss goals to work toward. Again, DASH dieting makes it much easier to lose weight because it puts the focus back on whole foods.

Fats and Their Impact on the Body

For a long time, fat was a bad word in the world of nutrition. Everyone told us to avoid fat in favor of low fat options, but now we know a lot more about it. We have discovered that fat is not all bad! In fact, some fats can lower your cholesterol and will actually lead to weight loss.

Fats have a number of essential functions in the human body.

➢ They provide energy
➢ They help maintain a healthy body temperature
➢ They help in the creation of new cells
➢ They protect organs
➢ They help absorb vitamins
➢ They produce hormones that help with essential bodily functions

The real trick is to balance the number of good fats with all of the other nutrition so that you are eating a balanced diet. This is where macros really come in handy!

Good Fats Versus Bad Fats

Fats are either healthy or harmful, depending on their composition. Unsaturated fats are healthy while saturated or trans fats are generally unhealthy. The difference is in their composition. Let's look at the science behind fat.

Fats are all comprised of carbon atoms which are bonded by hydrogen atoms. With saturated fats, the carbon atoms are covered (saturated) with hydrogen. This causes them to become solid at room temperature.

With unsaturated fat, there are fewer hydrogen atoms bound to carbon so they are liquid at room temperature.

With that being said, saturated fat is generally seen as unhealthy because it increases the amount of bad cholesterol in your body. It essentially raises your risk of heart disease and other serious conditions. You will find saturated fat in the following foods:

➢ Red meat (beef, lamb, pork)
➢ Poultry skin
➢ Whole fat dairy products
➢ Butter
➢ Eggs
➢ Processed oils

There is a lot of controversy surrounding saturated fats, but the truth is that it's really dependent on how much you abuse these foods. It's clear that a diet loaded with nothing but red meat will contribute to higher cholesterol levels. There are also some foods that are healthy, yet still contain saturated fat—like milk and cheese. DASH dieters will want to keep their consumption of red meat at a minimum.

No more than 5% of your calories should come from saturated fats. For example, if you are on a 2,000 calorie diet, then you should consume no more than 120 calories of saturated fat.

With that in mind, you should not remove all fats from your diet. Healthy fats are essential to our health. Don't replace those unhealthy fats with carbohydrates. That's what most people do. You should replace them with healthy fats.

The best part about the DASH diet is that it puts foods in front of us that are loaded in these healthy fats. It puts the right foods in front of us so we can avoid bad fats naturally.

Part 2

DASH Diet

and

Weight Loss

Chapter 6

DASH Dieting for Weight Loss

Incorporating the DASH diet into your everyday life can be quite a difficult task. That's why I recommend that you slowly transition your way into this new lifestyle. If you are looking to lose weight on this amazingly versatile dieting plan, then you will need to take a few additional steps.

Keep a Food Journal

You should record all of your daily eating habits in your food journal. Write down all of the foods that you eat throughout the day, and make a note if you happen to skip a meal. Record the calories for each meal and the activity you were doing while eating. The key to keeping a food journal is to write down every food you eat, including snacks. For some reason, a lot of people skip recording snacks or cheat meals. Snacking is probably the biggest challenge that we face when trying to lose weight because most snacking is done mindlessly. Keeping a food journal will force you to start thinking about everything that you eat.

Calculate Your Calories

Losing weight requires you to consume fewer calories than you burn on a daily basis, so you must keep track. You will have to start by figuring out your physical activity level, and then calculate how many calories you burn throughout the day. There are a lot of online calorie calculators that will give you this number. Now all you need to do is make sure that you consume fewer calories than you are burning. For example, a person who burns 2,500 calories per day should limit their intake to 2,000 calories if they want to lose weight.

Reduce the Consumption of Bad Fats

The DASH diet put emphasis on eating whole foods that contain healthy fats. It also gets you away from all of those unhealthy fats that are found in processed foods–saturated and trans fats. These two fats lead to higher cholesterol and will cause your blood pressure to be high. They will also cause you to gain weight. Reducing the consumption of bad fats will make it much easier to lose weight.

Consume Less Sugar

DASH dieters are encouraged to restrict their consumption of sugars. While I'm certainly not saying that completely restricting sweets is a bad thing, it is going to make it much more challenging for you to stay on the right path. I do not recommend that those new to this lifestyle completely restrict themselves. Instead, just make sure that you're being compliant 90% of the time. When you feel a sugar craving, try eating a piece of fruit rather than a donut. With that said, you do not have to restrict yourself entirely. You can have four to five servings of sweets every week without causing too much damage to your diet. Just make sure you count the sugar in your coffee and the jam you spread on your toast.

Lower Your Sodium Intake

The best way to accomplish this is to eat lean meats like poultry and fish rather than cooking up ham or bacon, both of which are loaded with sodium. The DASH diet limits sodium intake to anywhere between 1,500 mg to 2,300 mg, depending on which method you choose. You should also avoid adding salt to food when preparing it. There are some amazing seasonings that are completely free of sodium. Finally, make sure you read food labels to check for sodium in everything that you eat.

Eat More Fruits and Vegetables

You should be eating a lot of vegetables on the DASH diet – at least 5 servings per day to be exact. You'll also need to eat at least 4 servings of fruits every day. Remember that your vegetables do not have to be eaten on their own. You can add them to main dishes like stir-fry and brown rice. There is also a lot of different fruits that you can add to your diet, so make sure that you take advantage of the versatility that the DASH diet offers.

Eat More Whole Grains

It's important that you eat only whole grains while following the DASH diet. Experts agree that you should consume at least six servings of whole grains every day. This will make up most of your carb requirements for the day. For example, you can start with oatmeal, and then end your day with brown rice as a part of your dinner.

Advanced Changes That Will Lead to Optimal Weight Loss

We've gone over some of the basics, so now it's time to look at a few advanced strategies that you can include with the DASH diet that will boost your weight loss efforts.

Replace Unhealthy Snacks with Fruit

Pretty much every diet on the planet (ketogenic being an exception) tells you to do this because even though fruits are high in calories, they also contain essential vitamins and nutrients. So next time you are thinking about grabbing that snack cake from the vending machine, grab a piece of fruit instead. It is not only more nutritious, but it will satisfy your hunger for longer.

Practice Portion Control

Learn to eat smaller portions. There are several ways to do this, but the best is to never go back for seconds. You can also invest in smaller dishes so that you can't pile as much food on them. Also, don't eat while you are preoccupied. When we eat while watching television, our brain is too preoccupied to tell us that we're full, so we end up overeating as a result.

Eat Less at Night

You should eat less food at night so that your body is able to process it before you go to sleep. Now I will say that contrary to what many advocates might tell you, distributing calories throughout the day doesn't really make a difference as far as weight loss is concerned. Otherwise, intermittent fasting would not work. But I will say that if you can plan your larger meals directly after a workout or earlier in the day, then you'll make it easier on your body to process them.

Frequent Exercise Adds to Weight Loss

Combining exercise with the DASH diet will lead to some amazing results. Furthermore, it will decrease your risk for a number of diseases. Of course, exercise is completely optional, but it is the most effective method of enhancing your weight loss efforts.

Chapter 7
DASH Dieting Food Guide

This section is going to provide you with a general guideline to the foods that are allowed to be eaten on the DASH diet. You're going to want to focus on foods that are low in fat and cholesterol, mostly fruits and vegetables. Some of the other guidelines are to eat less sugar, salt, and red meat. We are basically cutting out a majority of the standard Western diet. Here is a look at some of the foods you should eat based on a 2,000 calorie diet.

Whole Grains (Seven Servings per Day)
You should always choose whole grain products over refined. They taste much better and are way healthier than their refined counterparts. Just be sure that you avoid those "whole grain snacks" like muffins and pancakes. It does little good to eat whole grains if you are loading them with refined sugar.

One serving of whole grain looks something like this:
- ➢ 1 Cup of sugar-free whole-grain cereal
- ➢ 1 Slice of whole grain bread
- ➢ ½ Cup oatmeal
- ➢ ½ Cup brown rice

Vegetables (Five Servings per Day)
This allowance is the bare minimum, but you can eat as many vegetables as you want. It doesn't really matter because vegetables are so low in calories and contain so many amazing nutrients.

One serving of vegetables looks something like this:

- ➢ 1 Cup of leafy vegetables (raw) like spinach or romaine lettuce
- ➢ ½ Cup cooked vegetables like carrots, broccoli, or squash
- ➢ 6 Oz. vegetable juice. Be sure to watch out for sodium and added sugar.

Fruit (Four Servings per Day)
You should always choose fresh or frozen fruit over their canned counterparts because sugar is usually added during the canning process. You should eat fruit as a snack or a replacement for dessert.

One serving of fruit looks something like this:

- ➢ 1 Piece of fruit like an apple, pear, or a banana
- ➢ ¼ Cup dried fruit like prunes, apricots, and mango
- ➢ ½ Cup fresh or frozen fruit like berries
- ➢ 6 Oz. fruit juice

Low-Fat Dairy Products (Three Servings per Day)
Always choose low-fat or fat-free dairy products over their full fat counterparts. Dairy contains a lot of essential nutrients, but it can also contain a lot of unhealthy fats. That's why we are going to opt for low fat options.

One serving of dairy looks something like this:

➢ 8 Oz. skim milk
➢ 1 Cup yogurt (pay attention to added sugar)
➢ 1 ½ Oz. Cheese

Lean Meats, Poultry, and Fish (Two Servings per Day)
Protein is an important part of a balanced diet. The problem is that the standard Western diet tends to put too much focus on meat. Furthermore, we are all used to unhealthy meats like hot dogs and bacon. The DASH diet calls for us to avoid those unhealthy choices and put our focus on leaner meats. Stay away from red meat, sausage, hamburgers, and cold-cuts.

One serving of meat looks something like this:
➢ 3 Oz. lean meat
➢ 3 Oz. chicken breast
➢ 3 Oz. turkey breast
➢ 3 Oz. fresh fish or tuna (avoid farm raised)
➢ 1 egg

Nuts and Seeds (Five Servings per Week)
Choose raw nuts and seed when possible. You do not want to eat those heavily salted nuts or those with added sugar. Nuts and seeds make an amazing snack because a small amount will satisfy your hunger for hours. Just be sure that you are following through with the DASH diet. Nuts and seeds that are heavily salted go against this diet.

One serving of nuts/seeds looks something like this:

➤ 1/3 Cup of nuts
➤ ½ Oz. seeds
➤ 2 Tbsp. peanut butter (no added sugar)

Fats and Oils (Two Servings per Day)
This is an important category because you should always choose healthy fats and oils over those refined, unhealthy options. Olive oil is a prime example of oil that is loaded with healthy fats. You can also use non-stick sprays since they contain no calories or fats. Finally, keep in mind that we are talking about oils here and not fats that occur naturally in foods like avocado and nuts.

One serving of oil looks something like this:

➤ 1 Tsp. olive oil

- ➢ 1 Tbsp. mayonnaise (low-fat)
- ➢ 2 Tbsp. salad dressing (low-fat)
- ➢ 1 Tsp. avocado oil

Sweet Treats (No More Than Three Servings per Week)
Sweet treats should be avoided for the most part, but one of the rules that I always encourage with all diets is that you do not become so restrictive that you set yourself up for failure. I teach a 90% compliance philosophy because it's healthier to be 90% compliant than not at all. As a result, you should limit your sweet treats to no more than three servings per week. Just remember that sugar added to your coffee counts, as does putting jam on your toast.

One serving of sweets looks something like this:

- ➢ 1 Tbsp. jam
- ➢ 1 Tbsp. sugar
- ➢ 8 Oz. sweet tea or lemonade

Alcoholic Beverages (No More Than One Drink per Day)
You should limit your alcohol intake to one drink per day. Just make sure that you avoid beverages that are high in sugar.

One serving looks like this:

- ➢ 5 Oz. wine
- ➢ 1.5 Oz. 80-proof whisky
- ➢ 12 Oz. beer

Chapter 8
Enhance Your Results with Exercise

We all know that exercise is healthy, but is it absolutely necessary in order to benefit from the DASH diet? Contrary to what many health advocates will tell you, going out of your way to exercise is not necessary for everyone. It depends on your own unique lifestyle. If you are a very active person or have a job that requires you to do a lot of manual labor, then chances are that you don't need to go out of your way to exercise. For example, if you work construction then going out of your way to exercise would be a bit repetitive since you get enough exercise working. However, if you work behind a desk then you probably need to take proactive steps to exercise.

The truth is that exercising, in combination with a healthy diet, will give you more energy and make you feel so much better! There are a lot of benefits to exercising that we're going to look at, but just remember that you should always take things slowly. Don't start intense workouts immediately. You will need to work your way into it slowly.

Exercise Helps Control Weight
Exercise will help you control your weight because of its powerful impact on your metabolism. You'll prevent excess

weight gain while also making it easier to lose weight in the first place. The truth is that while exercise is not a requirement in weight loss, it does make it so much easier.

You will burn calories when active. The more intense the activity, the more calories you will burn. While regular trips to the gym are highly beneficial, some people just can't afford to invest in the time required to be consistent, so my advice is to find ways to become more active that fit into your everyday life. I will walk through a number of these methods later in the book.

Exercise Combats Disease and Other Health Conditions

DASH dieting is designed to help prevent high blood pressure, so it's worth noting that exercise can actually enhance its effect. Exercise will also help prevent high blood pressure while also boosting your immune system. Furthermore, being active will boost your high-density lipoprotein (HDL) cholesterol which is also known as "good cholesterol." It also lowers those unhealthy triglycerides, known as "bad cholesterol."

Most doctors who prescribe DASH dieting will also encourage patients to exercise regularly. It's a powerful one-two punch!

Being active will also help prevent other health issues like stroke, metabolic syndrome, and even diabetes.

Exercise Improves Your Mood

If you find yourself needing an emotional lift then you need look no further than exercise. A short session in the gym or a 30-minute walk will improve your mood. When you're physically active, a number of chemicals are released in the brain. These chemicals will make you happier and more relaxed.

Furthermore, exercise will help you feel better about your appearance, so it boosts your confidence. Self-esteem is an important part of any lifestyle change. When you start growing confident in yourself, it becomes easier to stay consistent. You'll work harder on these improvements.

Exercise Is the Best Energy Booster!

You might wonder how being physically active will actually give you more energy. After all, exercising results in fatigue—at least that's what most people believe. Regular activity will provide a boost to your muscle growth, therefore giving you a significant metabolic boost. That's why we tend to have more energy after a big workout.

Exercising allows your tissues to soak in oxygen, which improves your blood flow. In short, it gives you much more energy throughout the day. That's why exercising in the morning is so beneficial.

Exercise Will Help You Sleep Better

If you are having trouble sleeping at night, then exercise is a solution! It helps you fall asleep faster and will even deepen your sleep. That's why people who have active jobs tend to get better sleep. Their schedule is consistent because they have no trouble falling asleep. They feel better and wake up earlier.

However, just make sure that you don't exercise too close to your bedtime. You will be too energized to fall asleep. Instead, an evening session should take place at least four hours prior to bed time.

Exercise Is a Fun and Social Experience

There are a number of ways that you can enjoy the benefits of physical activity, many of which are quite enjoyable. So don't limit yourself to spending hours on the treadmill or walking the same route every day. Try to engage in activities that you enjoy. Sports are a great way to get in your exercise while having a blast! Dance lessons are another!

Find activities that make you happy. That way you will be more likely to consistently follow through with them. If you get bored, then try something new.

How Often Should You Exercise?

First of all, you do not have to go out of your way to becoming more active. There are several ways that you can become more active. We're about to look at some of them, but for now, just understand that you will need to aim for at least 100 minutes of moderate activity every week.

Try to make small changes so that your body has a chance to adapt and then slightly increase your activity until you hit your final goal. I do encourage at least two 30-minute weight training sessions per week since building your muscle mass provides you with a permanent metabolic boost. In other words, the more muscles you have, the more calories your body will burn throughout the day.

Simple Ways to Become More Active

It's easy to get swept away by our everyday lives. We call it "fast-paced," but for many, this life of all work and no play is mostly sitting behind a desk. While it is definitely busy work-wise, it's not exactly an active lifestyle. That's why it's important to take steps to add physical activity into our everyday life.

The following methods are an easy way to become more active in your everyday life. You'll start to become more mindful about these little things and turn everyday tasks into mini-workouts. You will be amazed at how much better you feel.

Walk More

Rather than driving two blocks to pick up the latest magazine from the magazine stand, walk those two blocks. This one simple decision will get you a 10 to 15 minute workout without having to go out of your way. You can also go for walks while chatting with your friend. Whatever it takes to walk more rather than just sitting around will help you become more active.

Take the Stairs Rather Than the Elevator
Did you know that just 5 minutes of walking up the stairs can burn as many as 150 calories? If you work on an upper floor, then start walking up the stairs rather than taking the elevator. This is a small change where you don't really have to go out of your way to become more active. If you do this 5 times per week you have the potential to burn over 700 calories!

Clean More
Not only is having a clean house an amazing feeling, cleaning can burn up to 200 calories an hour. You should clean for at least one hour per week. Having a clean home is motivational, and you will be killing two birds with one stone. Your home will be clean, and you'll be burning 200 calories every week with no extra effort.

Use a Basket for Shopping Whenever Possible
If you are just making a short trip into the store, then you should use a basket rather than a cart. It's automatic for us to reach for a cart no matter what, but when you use a basket,

you're getting in an automatic weightlifting session. It can actually add up to quite the workout.

Park Further Away

While everyone else is fighting tooth and nail for those close parking spots, start parking further away so that you are forced to walk further. You will actually save a lot of time that you would have wasted looking for a close parking spot. Additionally, you will get in a mini workout by walking further.

Start Playing with Your Pet

It goes without saying but if you have a dog, then you will have to go on frequent walks. So why not take it a step further by playing with your furry friend? Dogs are full of energy and will happily play games. You can get in a good workout while your dog stays happy! You can do the same thing with your cat. They also love to play, but you'll usually have to initiate it. My point is that playing with your pet is an amazingly fun way to stay active.

Get Up At Least Once Every Hour

It's easy to lose track of time while working behind a desk, so set an alarm to remind yourself to get up every hour. You should walk around or stretch for a minimum of two minutes before returning to your work. There are also programs like Break Pal that not only alert you when it's time to stand, but they give you a few simple tasks to perform before sitting back down.

The point that I am trying to make here is that small additions to your routine can make a huge difference. These changes will make it so that you don't have to go out of your way to exercise to become more active. Once you establish new habits, they become an automatic part of your everyday routine.

Exercises to Enhance the DASH Diet

For those of you who want to enhance the DASH diet even further, then you will want to include a few exercises into your daily routine. We'll look at some of the best workouts to include while DASH dieting.

Aerobic Exercise

Aerobic exercises will improve your circulation and help lower your blood pressure, making them the absolute best form of exercise to combine with DASH dieting. Additionally, it will help control how strongly your heart pumps blood and reduce the risk of type-2 diabetes. Even if you already have diabetes, aerobic exercise will help your body control glucose levels.

Frequency: You should aim to exercise at least 120 minutes per week.

Examples of Aerobic Exercise

- ➢ Walking
- ➢ Running
- ➢ Swimming
- ➢ Cycling
- ➢ Sports
- ➢ Jump Rope

Strength Training

Strength training will have a more specific effect on the composition of your body. Individuals who are hauling around a lot of excess fat will find strength training to be quite beneficial to their weight loss efforts. Additionally, studies have shown that the combination of aerobic exercise and strength training actually lowers bad cholesterol levels while raising good cholesterol levels.

Frequency: Strength training workouts should be performed at least two days a week, making sure to rest for at least one day in between.

Examples of Strength Training Exercises

- ➢ Weightlifting
- ➢ Curling
- ➢ Resistance band workouts
- ➢ Push-ups
- ➢ Squats
- ➢ Pull-ups

Stretching and Balance Exercises
While flexibility workouts do not necessarily contribute to hearth health, they do enable you to stay flexible and free from joint pain. They help enhance your other workouts by keeping you from cramping and other muscular issues. That flexibility is an essential part of being able to consistently perform aerobic and resistance based exercises. By having a good musculoskeletal foundation, you will be able to keep doing the exercises that improve the health of your heart.

Frequency: Daily before and after all workouts.

Examples of Stretching and Balancing Exercises

➤ Yoga
➤ Tai Chi
➤ Stretches

Chapter 9

Calorie Needs for Weight Loss

This is an important topic for those of you looking to lose weight. While the DASH diet is not necessarily designed for weight loss, eating whole foods and vegetables will make weight loss much easier to achieve. We're going to take a closer look at calories and how they affect our weight.

On average, men will need to consume no more than 2,000 calories in order to lose weight while women will need to consume no more than 1,500 calories. But the actual numbers vary depending on a number of factors. Age, height, weight, and activity levels play a pivotal role in determining your exact calorie needs. Let's dive deeper into this important topic!

What Are Calories Exactly?

Calories are a measurement for energy that our body uses to fuel itself. We normally see this unit displayed on food and beverages. The human body uses calories to perform everyday tasks to keep up alive. Any excess energy is stored as fat so that it can be released when needed. In order to get our body to burn this fat, we have to consume fewer calories than our body burns. That forces it to use all of the excess stored energy.

You can find several online calorie calculators that will give you an idea as to how many calories your body burns. This is based on weight, age, gender, and how active you are. I highly recommend that you plug your numbers into a calculator to set your calorie goals.

Reduce Calorie Intake Without Starving Yourself

We lose weight when we consume fewer calories than we burn, so cutting calories is essential to weight loss. DASH dieting makes it much easier to lower your calorie intake because your focus will be on whole foods. In short, you can eat more whole foods and stay under your calorie count. On the other hand, processed foods tend to be loaded in calories and do not provide the same nutritional value.

The reason so many people fail to lose weight is because they end up trying to starve themselves. One of the most important things to remember is that you cannot win a fight against your biology. If your body is hungry, your biological urge to overeat is going to eventually overwhelm you. It might take weeks, or even months, but it will eventually win.

That's why it's important to make lifestyle changes that will help you stay at a calorie deficit while also ensuring that you stay satisfied. Here are some amazing lifestyle changes that you can make that will help you control calories while ensuring that you are not starving yourself.

Eat More Protein

Consuming more protein will reduce your appetite while cutting down on your cravings. Furthermore, it will even increase the number of calories you burn. With the DASH diet, we're aiming to reduce the amount of red meats that we consume, but we can find protein from a number of different sources.

With weight loss, protein is king when it comes to nutrients. Adding more of this essential nutrient to your diet makes it much easier to lose weight. Plus, you can create some delicious protein-based meals.

Protein is proven to increase your metabolic rate while also curbing your appetite. The real challenge is finding the healthiest foods to provide you with protein. You're not going to be able to scarf down hamburgers all day long and lose weight. However, adding more fish and lean meats to your lifestyle will enhance your weight loss efforts.

You can make an effort to add healthy proteins to your diet, and it will reduce the amount of calories you consume because it satisfies you for longer.

Stop Drinking Your Calories

Any calories that you gain through beverages are a complete waste. You are getting calories with little to no nutritional value. So stay away from sodas and fruit juice. If you start tracking when you eat and drink, you will be astonished at how many calories are wasted through beverages. It's no wonder that so many people have trouble losing weight!

Our brain does not register liquid calories like it does solid foods. Even though we are getting energy through liquids, our body will still crave those solid foods because it needs the nutrients. In other words, our body will not compensate for that sugary beverage by having us eat less, so those calories are a complete waste.

In fact, there are a number of studies that show a direct link between obesity and sugary beverages. Of course, we don't really need a study to show us just how unhealthy soda can be. They do so much more damage than just weight gain. They wreak utter havoc on your body! They are disastrous to our metabolic health and increase our risk for a number of diseases.

It's okay to eat fruits and consume other foods that contain natural sugars, but those drinks that are loaded in refined sugars are quite disastrous. Fruit juice is also just as bad as soda. Fruits should be consumed in their whole form. We do not need these drinks, and avoiding them will have a positive impact on our health.

Drink More Water

The more water we drink, the easier it will be to lose weight. This is probably the simplest and most effective starting point for your journey towards a healthier life. While there is a formula for determining the exact amount of water you should drink per day, I recommend that you start with 68 ounces. Drinking this much water daily will make you burn around 100 extra calories.

Timing is also essential. For instance, if you drink a glass of water before eating a meal then you will eat less. When you combine this with a healthy plan like the DASH diet, you will experience some amazing results. In fact, you can lose up to 40% more weight by consuming the right amount of water every day.

Caffeinated beverages will also contribute positively to your health as long as you don't add sugar. That means you can enjoy your coffee and green tea as long as you leave out the refined sugar. It will actually boost your metabolism.

Become More Active

If we try restricting calories without becoming more active, our body will actually start to slow down in an attempt to store more energy. Therefore, it burns less so that it can store more. This is the exact opposite of what we want.

I'm not saying that you have to go out of your way to exercise every day. On the contrary, I have shown you several small changes that you can make to become more active. Those are enough to offset this problem. However, adding strength training and aerobic exercises will enhance your calorie efficiency even further.

Reduce Wasteful Carbs

Cutting back on the number of carbs you eat will help improve your fat burning potential. It also helps you consume fewer calories because fewer carbs lead to a reduction in appetite. Therefore, it will automatically lower your intake of calories.

You don't have to completely restrict your calories while on the DASH diet, but you should make sure that you're getting quality carbs like whole wheat and other single ingredient foods. When you stick to whole foods, the composition of your diet is less important.

Again, avoiding sugars and other processed foods will help you naturally avoid these wasteful carbs. Your focus should be on whole foods.

The Bottom Line on Calories

The number of calories you need per day will depend on your unique lifestyle. Individuals who are more active will need more calories. Factors like age, height, and current weight also play an important role.

Reducing calorie intake does not mean that you should starve yourself. It means that you need to make sure that the calories you're getting are not wasted. For example, vegetables are loaded in nutrients, but they have a low calorie count.

Chapter 10

Become a Master Meal Planner

Many people are intimidated by meal planning, seeing it as an overwhelming task. The problem is that we tend to see meal planning from the back end. We imagine this huge binder organized with tabs pointing us to specific recipes. We imagine the pantry full of foods that are just waiting to be prepared. When all of this is put in front of someone new to meal planning, of course they're going to become anxious. From the outside, it looks so complicated.

I am going to lay out a system for meal planning that is extremely simple. It can be broken down into three steps— recipe selection, shopping, and prepping. I know it sounds obvious, but there are critical points that need to be made during each step. Effective meal planning will save you money and is an essential step to living a healthier lifestyle.

By the time you are finished reading this chapter, you will have a detailed blueprint for creating your own meal plan.

Before we get started, let me explain exactly what meal planning is so that we're all on the same page.

Meal planning is the process of planning out your meals for an entire week at a time rather than waiting until you're hungry to plan for dinner. What makes it so valuable is that you can focus your shopping to very specific ingredients rather than randomly throwing items in the cart.

Scheduling a day for planning is also an important step to take because you should strive to be consistent. I like to do my meal planning on Friday so that I can use the weekend for shopping and prepping my meals. But you can choose whatever day works best for your lifestyle.

With that being said, meal planning is not some magical solution that will solve all of your problems. It is a powerful tool, but it's not going to "change your life." It is designed to solve specific problems that are associated with dieting. You will also have to tailor this process to fit your unique lifestyle.

Don't let meal planning intimidate you. I'm not asking you to fill a huge binder with a month's worth of recipes. You will just write down your plan in a planner or stick it to the front of your refrigerator. You can even hang a whiteboard in your kitchen with your plan in full view.

Another important note is that you do not necessarily have to plan for all home-cooked meals. You can plan for eating out as well. I do not believe in being too restrictive. It's important that you enjoy the choices you make. If you don't enjoy it, then you will eventually give up.

What Exactly Do You Need?

You'll need to define the reason why you are interested in meal planning. For those of you reading this book, you're planning ahead to make it easier to stay on track with the DASH diet. Knowing why will help you understand exactly what you need. What are some other goals that you have?

➢ Do you want to save money?
➢ Are you looking to add variety?
➢ Do you want to prevent wasting food?

Burnout is a very real factor to consider, so those of you who are new to this program should choose a few goals that really matter to them. Then always keep these goals in the back of your mind so that you can stay motivated.

Step 1: Choose Your Recipes

This step requires you to know exactly why you are planning your meals. It pretty much sets the entire process in motion. For DASH dieting, we're looking for recipes that are based around whole foods. You are not going to just choose a bunch of random recipes and hope for the best. In fact, I think you should spend a week or two carefully choosing recipes. Don't worry because I am going to provide you with a meal plan in this book so that you can start DASH dieting right away.

The first thing you will want to do is choose how many meals per day you are going to plan for. DASH dieting requires a minimum of three meals per day with a snack somewhere between meals. But you can start slow. Plan for three meals per week, and once you get used to planning for that, start planning for five meals. Keep gradually increasing the number of meals you plan for until you are planning a full week at a time.

Hone it all in even further. What will you need to do on the nights you plan to cook? For instance, do you have a busy night planned? If so, then a slow cooker recipe might be your best bet. You might also need to plan something large enough so that you have leftovers for lunch.

Now you are ready to look for recipes. You can do a quick Google search and find DASH dieting recipes. Make sure that these recipes are low in sodium and that they are based on whole foods.

You should choose recipes that will leave you with leftovers. They are the meals that keep on giving!

Another good rule of thumb is to plan for recipes that you know while adding one new recipe every week. This is what experienced meal planners do because it adds variety and keeps your meals interesting. There are certain recipes that you will know by heart, but it's important that you learn new ones as you continue on your journey.

You should try to choose recipes that are based on common ingredients so that you are able to shop more efficiently. Another good strategy is to keep track of ingredients that are leftover from the previous week and plan for recipes that use them. This is a pro move that will help you avoid wasting food. It also saves money!

Only cook meals that you want to eat. It might sound obvious, but you would be surprised at how many people will cook meals that do not excite them just because they are on a diet. Make sure that you're excited about meal time!

Step 2: Create a Smart Shopping List

By this point, you should have a list of recipes that you want to prepare. Now you just need to get the ingredients to make them! This is the step that intimidates most people, so I'm going to lay it out in two easy actions so that you don't get overwhelmed. This doesn't take a long time at all. Doing it just one time will teach you everything you need to know. After that, you'll be an expert in creating a shopping list.

The first action is to create a master ingredient list. This is not your shopping list, but it will eventually lead you in that direction. You simple go through each recipe and make a list of all ingredients. Then go through your kitchen and mark off any ingredients that you already have. You will be left with a list that can easily be transformed into a grocery list.

When you choose recipes that are based on things you already have in your pantry, then you'll be crossing a lot of items off of the master list. However, you can leave pantry items on the list so that you can restock it.

The second action is to actually make the shopping list. You could theoretically take your ingredient list into the supermarket to use as a shopping list, but I'm going to show you a much better way. Rewriting this list allows you to organize it better.

Group ingredients together by how they will be found in the supermarket. You should take it a step further by placing those groups in order based on how the store is laid out. For instance, you would want the frozen foods at the end of the list so that you pick them up last. If you plan on having the store slice your meat, then you can swing by that department first.

Step 3: Prep for the Coming Week

For most people, spending one hour on Sunday prepping is going to be the best approach. You should have all of the ingredients at this point, so let's focus on getting those meals ready to cook. This step is essential to long-term success on any dieting plan because there will be times during the week when you don't feel like prepping. So let's get it all done at once!

You will be chopping everything up and putting it away so that all you need to do is mix everything together when it comes time to cook. At this stage, your planning will start to transform into meals. The exact steps here depend on the recipes you have chosen, but the idea is to get everything possible prepped for the coming week. Here are some examples:

- ➢ Dicing onions
- ➢ Washing fresh veggies
- ➢ Cook meats for stews
- ➢ Dice up garlic

Do everything you can now so that when it comes time to actually cook the meal, you will be prepared for it.

Practice Makes Perfect!

Don't stop now! Keep up the momentum. Meal planning is one of the most effective ways to follow through with DASH dieting. The reason most people eat unhealthy foods is because they are more convenient. Planning ensures that your meals are all convenient, so you are less likely to fail.

Planning gets easier over time. The more you do it, the better you will become. Keep it up!

Chapter 11

Keep a Food Journal to Enhance Weight Loss

Keeping a food journal is an amazingly powerful tool that will help you achieve health goals that once seems far out of reach. While it's not a requirement of DASH dieting, journaling is going to give you more control and make it so much easier to find success.

Gaining control over your diet will have a positive effect on your health and lifestyle. Journaling also comes with a lot of other benefits. For instance, if you have digestive problems then a journal will help you track down what foods are causing them.

For the purpose of DASH dieting, it will give you an overview of the foods you're eating to make sure you're getting in the right nutrients.

Food Journaling: Phase 1–Meal Tracking

Step 1: Set Up Your Diary.
The easiest way to set up a food journal is to utilize the latest technology to assist you. Download a food journaling app on your phone. These apps will make it easy to track everything that goes into your body.

If you are an advocate of writing things down, then you can purchase a notebook and keep track of everything you eat. Search Google for some sample food journal pages to use as a reference.

Step 2: Record Everything

This is a step that so many people get wrong. It's easy to forget writing down that drink you had with lunch or that small candy bar you cheated with as a snack. I know that it's hard to record our failures, but you must make sure you include those in your journal. Understanding why we are making mistakes is the only way to avoid them in the future.

You'll want to be as specific as possible. Break down complicated recipes into ingredients so that you can see the exact food groups. For instance, rather than writing down "turkey sandwich," you should separate it into categories like bread, turkey, and condiments. All foods should be broken down this way.

You must record all beverages as well, including water, so that you know you're getting enough water every day. You must drink enough water to stay hydrated every day. This is a step that so many people ignore.

Step 3: Be as Accurate as Possible

When tracking your calorie intake, you have to write down the quantities of food that you're eating. You might need to invest in some measuring cups and a food scale.

You can also spend a couple of weeks documenting your normal diet before swapping over to the DASH diet. That way, you have a visual reference for the changes that you need to make. Then you can determine whether each portion is too big or too small and make adjustments as necessary.

You will continue to measure your food using measuring cups and food scales. It's essential that you be as accurate as possible. Estimating portion sizes is not quite accurate enough because then you could be wrong on your calorie intake. The only time you will have to estimate portion sizes is when eating out or with foods that are difficult to weigh.

You'll also want to keep a close eye on the calories with each meal. Track calories for all ingredients, each meal, and also include a daily total. This makes it easier to control how many calories you are putting into your body. If a recipe is putting you over the top, then you can reduce an ingredient to get back on track.

One of the best features about using a journaling app is that it will automatically add up your calories. Plus, some apps will even provide nutritional information for certain foods for you, so you don't have to do any additional research.

Again, you will start out by calculating your normal calorie count, and then use that as an indicator of which areas you need to improve on. Keep in mind that 500 calories results in 1 pound on average. For instance, if you overeat by 500 calories then you will gain 1 pound and vice versa—if you eat 500 calories less then you will lose 1 pound.

Step 4: Document Date, Time, and Location

This is an essential part of finding patterns in your eating habits. If you are trying to make changes to your lifestyle, then you are going to want to find out what eating habits are dragging you down. Some people tend to eat more calories while watching television. Others will eat healthy until they eat out where they will then throw all of their good habits out of the window.

Write down the exact time. Don't use vague descriptions like "afternoon snack." You should also record the activity while you were eating. If you were watching television during dinner, then be sure to write that down. If you were in a hurry, note that as well.

Step 5: Record How You Felt

Another powerful part of keeping a food journal is that it can show you the role that your mood is having on your eating habits. You should be able to look back and see what your mood was when you were eating certain foods.

A lot of the times, people will eat when they're bored and not because they're hungry. When we start becoming aware of this problem, we stop eating based on emotion. The key is to only eat when you're hungry.

Take notes about your mood when you were eating when recording foods on your list. You should also wait at least 20 minutes after each meal and then take a note about how you feel. Are you satisfied? Do you feel sleepy? Do you have energy?

By this point, you should have a list of foods, calories, and your mood both before and after you eat. This journal will become such a powerful tool on your journey to living a healthier life. Remember that emotional eating is unhealthy because it usually causes you to eat large portions of food. Plus, you might be turning to comfort foods when you're emotional. The only way you will know for sure is by documenting everything you eat.

Food Journaling: Phase 2–Analyze Your Diet

Step 1: Look for Patterns
Pay attention to potential patterns in your eating habits. After a few weeks of tracking in your journal, you will be able to spot patterns. We all have certain patterns that we follow.

We don't even realize it! So pinpointing these will help you avoid bad eating habits. Answer these questions:

> What are the exact patterns you follow when eating?
> Are those patterns related to your mood?
> Which foods leave you satisfied?
> Which meals leave you hungry?
> What was your mood when you overate?

Step 2: Count the Number of Snacks You Eat
Most people are surprised by how many snacks they eat on a daily basis. It's easy to fall into the habit of snacking far too often. A cookie or two here and a bag of chips there can add up to a lot of wasted calories. When are you snacking? The Western diet usually follows the habit of snacking on junk food while watching television.

If you want to live a healthier life, then you must develop healthier eating habits. Achieving these healthier eating habits starts with identifying them. Use your food journal to assess where you can improve your snacking. In many cases, it only takes very small changes to make a huge difference.

Start choosing healthier snacks. Try stepping away from the television while you snack or make sure you only keep a small amount of food within reach.

The goal to healthy eating is to only eat when you're hungry.

Step 3: Compare Weekdays to Weekend Days

Work and school have a significant effect on our eating habits. This effect is not always so obvious until we see it in writing. This is why a food journal has such a huge impact on most people. For instance, most people make unhealthy choices on weekdays because they lack the time to eat. But these same people might make healthy choices on weekends because they have more time. We all tend to base a lot of our decisions on convenience rather than health.

Do you eat out more during the week? If so, then you should prepare meals in advance so that you have something convenient to grab and heat up. This information should be used to help you plan your meals in advance. Once you understand why you are making unhealthy choices, you can start taking proactive steps to develop better habits.

Step 4: Study Your Emotional Connection with Food

Take notes in regards to the emotional connection you have with food. Figure out what life situations are influencing your eating habits on any given day. There could be patterns in food choices based on your emotional state.

> ➢ Do you eat more when you're lonely?
> ➢ Are you making unhealthy food choices because you're stressed and need comfort food?
> ➢ Are you having a midnight snack because you can't sleep?

The more you understand about yourself, the better choices you will make. When it comes to planning your diet, you need to account for the role that your mood plays.

If there an issue with overeating when you're upset, then you should try engaging in another activity to counter that stress. You could meditate or engage in some kind of physical activity.

Certain foods can actually lead to negative emotions, so you need to pinpoint these as well. One example is that drinking too much coffee in the morning can make you feel jittery.

Step 5: Find Food Intolerances
By this point, you should have recorded a lot of information about your eating habits, so now you should go through your journal and identify foods that you are negatively impacting your body. Your journal might reveal that you're lactose intolerant so you know to avoid dairy products.

Certain foods might give you a tummy ache or make you feel bloated. You can identify these as well so that you know to avoid them in the future.

Will a Food Journal Actually Help?

Whether you are trying to lose weight or are just trying to make healthier choices, the DASH diet is an amazing long-term solution. Keeping a food journal will help boost its effectiveness. Not only will a food journal help, it will become the most powerful tool at your disposal.

Journaling Will Help You Lose Weight

Food journaling will show you all of those unhealthy eating habits that you've developed. In most cases, those habits are what cause people to struggle with weight loss, so by understanding them, we are able to start taking steps to thwart their impact. You'll be able to bring a healthy snack to work so that you can avoid the dreaded vending machine.

You'll Define Food Intolerances

Food journaling helps you spot patterns in foods that might be making you feel poorly after eating them. We all have different reactions to food, and these reactions can happen hours after we eat. Journaling gives you a written record of how your body reacts to food.

Food Journals Assist in Portion Control

This might be the single most important habit to develop when trying to lead a healthier life. You must learn to control how much you eat. Portion control is extremely difficult in today's world, but a food journal will help you understand how much you are eating at every meal. If you find that you're eating too much at night then you can make minor adjustments to the way you eat throughout the day. For example, you might consider including a late afternoon snack so that you don't go into dinner starving.

Journaling Improves Your Nutrition

Keeping track of your meals will reveal so much more than simple calorie intake. It will show you if you're eating the right types of foods and the number of nutrients you are getting in your diet. If your diet is too rich in carbohydrates, then you might be missing out on important fats. Or you could be slacking on fruit and overeating meat. The only way you will know for sure is by keeping a food journal.

A Food Journal Helps You Find Triggers

This is why you want to track your mood before and after each meal. Having these things on record will give you an idea of certain triggers that you might possess. For instance, some people find themselves reaching for a candy bar at work when they are dealing with a stressful deadline. This is an item that could be identified with a journal. Then that individual could find another way to cope with the stress, like getting up and walking around the office.

Final Thoughts

Although DASH dieting was designed to help lower blood pressure, it is also an effective weight-loss tool. It's one of the best dieting plans in the world because of its focus on whole foods. That focus makes it easy to stay on track for the long-term. In short, you will have a much easier time of achieving long-term success following the DASH diet than any other diet.

The final sections of this book are going to show you a four-week meal plan that you can follow to help you get started. You will find out that the foods included in the DASH dieting meal plan include a ton of tasty recipes.

DASH dieting is recommended by:

> ➢ The National Heart, Lung, and Blood Institute
> ➢ The American Heart Association
> ➢ The Dietary Guidelines for Americans

Make sure you're giving your body exactly what it needs to thrive.

Part 3

Four-Week

Meal Plan

Meal Plan Introduction

The best way to help you get on the right path is to provide you with a four-week meal plan. This is going to make your journey towards a healthier life much easier. As you know, my goal is to provide you with everything you need to make your transition to the DASH diet as easy as possible. Here are a few notes about the following meal plan.

1. Some meals in this plan will leave you with leftovers, so you don't have to cook every day. This can be a lifesaver for those of you who are constantly busy.

2. You should always track your daily calories and make sure you are under your recommended count if your goal is to lose weight. You will only lose weight if you are at a calorie deficit.

3. Being active is an essential part of living a healthier life. However, if you are physically active throughout the day, then you do not necessarily have to follow through with an exercise plan.

Week 1

Monday

Breakfast: Baked Eggs with Cheesy Hash

Snack: ½ Banana, Palm Full of Nuts

Lunch: Tuna Salad Sandwich

Snack: ½ Banana, Palm Full of Nuts

Dinner: Penne Pasta with Spinach and Bacon

Dessert: Yogurt with Nuts and Raspberries

Tuesday

Breakfast: Sausage Egg Muffins

Snack: ½ Banana

Lunch: Penne Pasta with Spinach and Bacon (leftover from Monday)

Snack: ½ Banana

Dinner: Smoked Salmon Fried Rice

Dessert: Yogurt with Nuts and Raspberries

Wednesday

Breakfast: Sweet Potato Breakfast Bake

Snack: 1 Apple

Lunch: White Bean and Avocado Salad

Snack: Palm full of nuts

Dinner: Turkey Veggie Meatload Cups

Dessert: Fig and Honey Yogurt

Thursday

Breakfast: Ultimate Breakfast Roll Ups

Snack: ½ Banana, Palm Full of Nuts

Lunch: Old Fashioned Potato Salad

Snack: ½ Banana, Palm Full of Nuts

Dinner: Turkey Veggie Meatload Cups (leftover from Wednesday)

Dessert: Banana Ice Cream (Frozen banana put through food processor)

Friday

Breakfast: Yogurt with Nuts and Raspberries

Snack: 1 Apple

Lunch: Black Bean Chili

Snack: Palm Full of Nuts

Dinner: Baked Honey Mustard Chicken

Dessert: Grape Ice Cream (frozen grapes put through food processor)

Saturday

Breakfast: Carrot Cake Oatmeal

Snack: ½ Banana

Lunch: Baked Honey Mustard Chicken (leftover from Friday)

Snack: ½ Banana

Dinner: Black Bean Chili (leftover from Friday)

Dessert: Yogurt with Nuts and Raspberries

Sunday

Breakfast: Peanut-Butter Cinnamon Toast

Snack: ½ Grapefruit

Lunch: Curried Cauliflower Steaks with Red Rice

Snack: ½ Grapefruit

Dinner: Curried Cauliflower Steaks with Red Rice (leftover from lunch)

Dessert: Banana Ice Cream (frozen bananas put through food processor)

Week 2

Monday
Breakfast: Baked Eggs with Cheesy Hash

Snack: ½ Banana, Palm Full of Nuts

Lunch: Tuna Salad Sandwich

Snack: ½ Banana, Palm Full of Nuts

Dinner: Smoked Salmon Fried Rice

Dessert: Yogurt with Nuts and Raspberries

Tuesday
Breakfast: Sweet Potato Breakfast Bake

Snack: 1 Apple

Lunch: Stuffed Sweet Potato with Hummus Dressing

Snack: Palm full of nuts

Dinner: Smoked Salmon Fried Rice (leftover from Monday)

Dessert: Yogurt with Nuts and Raspberries

Wednesday
Breakfast: Sausage Egg Muffins

Snack: ½ Banana

Lunch: Stuffed Sweet Potato with Hummus Dressing (leftover from Tuesday)

Snack: ½ Banana

Dinner: Ginger Mahi Mahi

Dessert: Fig and Honey Yogurt

Thursday

Breakfast: Peanut-Butter Cinnamon Toast

Snack: ½ Banana, Palm Full of Nuts

Lunch: Veggie-Hummus Sandwich

Snack: ½ Banana, Palm Full of Nuts

Dinner: Creamy Fettuccine with Brussels Sprouts and Mushrooms

Dessert: Yogurt with Nuts and Raspberries

Friday

Breakfast: Carrot Cake Oatmeal

Snack: 1 Apple

Lunch: Creamy Fettuccine with Brussels Sprouts and Mushrooms (leftover from Thursday)

Snack: Palm full of nuts

Dinner: Garlic Chicken with Orzo Noodles

Dessert: Grape Ice Cream (frozen grapes put through food processor)

Saturday

Breakfast: Yogurt with Nuts and Raspberries

Snack: ½ Banana

Lunch: Chorizo-Spiced Chopped Veggie Salad

Snack: ½ Banana

Dinner: Baked Tilapia

Dessert: Yogurt with Nuts and Raspberries

Sunday

Breakfast: Ultimate Breakfast Rollup

Snack: ½ Grapefruit

Lunch: Heart-Healthy Chicken Stew

Snack: ½ Grapefruit

Dinner: Heart-Healthy Chicken Stew (leftover from lunch)

Dessert: Banana Ice Cream (frozen bananas put through food processor)

Week 3

Monday

Breakfast: Yogurt with Nuts and Raspberries

Snack: ½ Banana, Palm Full of Nuts

Lunch: Spicy Avocado

Snack: ½ Banana, Palm Full of Nuts

Dinner: Quinoa Meatless Balls

Dessert: Fig and Honey Yogurt

Tuesday

Breakfast: Sausage Egg Muffins

Snack: ½ Banana

Lunch: Quinoa Meatless Balls (leftover from Monday)

Snack: ½ Banana

Dinner: Roasted New Potatoes

Dessert: Yogurt with Nuts and Raspberries

Wednesday

Breakfast: Sweet Potato Breakfast Bake

Snack: 1 Apple

Lunch: Veggie-Hummus Sandwich

Snack: Palm Full of Nuts

Dinner: Quinoa and Black Beans

Dessert: Fig and Honey Yogurt

Thursday

Breakfast: Ultimate Breakfast Roll Ups

Snack: ½ Banana, Palm Full of Nuts

Lunch: Old Fashioned Potato Salad

Snack: ½ Banana, Palm Full of Nuts

Dinner: Quinoa and Black Beans (leftover from Wednesday)

Dessert: Yogurt with Nuts and Raspberries

Friday

Breakfast: Baked Eggs with Cheesy Hash

Snack: 1 Apple

Lunch: Old Fashioned Potato Salad

Snack: Palm full of nuts

Dinner: Lemon-Garlic Shrimp over Orzo with Zucchini

Dessert: Grape Ice Cream (frozen grapes put through food processor)

Saturday

Breakfast: Carrot Cake Oatmeal

Snack: ½ Banana

Lunch: Lemon-Garlic Shrimp over Orzo with Zucchini (leftover from Friday)

Snack: ½ Banana

Dinner: Penne Pasta with Spinach and Bacon

Dessert: Yogurt with Nuts and Raspberries

Sunday

Breakfast: Peanut-Butter Cinnamon Toast

Snack: ½ Grapefruit

Lunch: Braised Balsamic Chicken

Snack: ½ Grapefruit

Dinner: Baked Tilapia

Dessert: Banana Ice Cream (frozen bananas put through food processor)

Week 4

Monday

Breakfast: Sausage Egg Muffins

Snack: ½ Banana, Palm Full of Nuts

Lunch: Chorizo-Spiced Chopped Veggie Salad

Snack: ½ Banana, Palm Full of Nuts

Dinner: Braised Balsamic Chicken

Dessert: Yogurt with Nuts and Raspberries

Tuesday

Breakfast: Carrot Cake Oatmeal

Snack: 1 Apple

Lunch: Braised Balsamic Chicken (leftover from Monday)

Snack: Palm Full of Nuts

Dinner: Ginger Mahi Mahi

Dessert: Yogurt with Nuts and Raspberries

Wednesday

Breakfast: Baked Eggs with Cheesy Hash

Snack: ½ Banana

Lunch: Split Pea Soup

Snack: ½ Banana

Dinner: Ginger Mahi Mahi (leftover from Tuesday)

Dessert: Fig and Honey Yogurt

Thursday

Breakfast: Peanut-Butter Cinnamon Toast

Snack: ½ Banana, Palm Full of Nuts

Lunch: Split Pea Soup (leftover from Wednesday)

Snack: ½ Banana, Palm Full of Nuts

Dinner: Stuffed Sweet Potato with Hummus Dressing

Dessert: Yogurt with Nuts and Raspberries

Friday

Breakfast: Yogurt with Nuts and Raspberries

Snack: 1 Apple

Lunch: Tuna Salad Sandwich

Snack: Palm full of nuts

Dinner: White Bean Chicken Chili

Dessert: Grape Ice Cream (frozen grapes put through food processor)

Saturday
Breakfast: Sweet Potato Breakfast Bake

Snack: ½ Banana

Lunch: White Bean Chicken Chili (leftover from Friday)

Snack: ½ Banana

Dinner: Spicy Black-Eyed Peas

Dessert: Yogurt with Nuts and Raspberries

Sunday
Breakfast: Ultimate Breakfast Rollup

Snack: ½ Grapefruit

Lunch: Mediterranean Chicken with Orzo Salad

Snack: ½ Grapefruit

Dinner: Curried Cauliflower Steaks with Red Rice

Dessert: Banana Ice Cream (frozen bananas put through food processor)

Part 4

Recipes

List of Recipes

Recipes

Baked Eggs with Cheesy Hash

Ingredients

- ✓ 5 Oz. diced zucchini
- ✓ 6 Oz. chopped cauliflower
- ✓ ½ Red bell pepper, medium and diced
- ✓ 1 Tbsp. melted coconut oil
- ✓ 1 Tsp. smoked paprika
- ✓ 1 Tsp. onion powder
- ✓ 1 Tsp. garlic powder
- ✓ ¼ Cup Mexican blend shredded cheese
- ✓ ½ Avocado, medium
- ✓ 3 Large eggs
- ✓ 1 Tbsp. sliced jalapenos
- ✓ 3 Tbsp. cotija cheese
- ✓ 2 Tsp. Tajin seasoning

Directions

1. Preheat oven to 400 degrees.

2. Line a baking sheet with foil and spread zucchini, cauliflower, and red peppers evenly into baking pan. Then drizzle it with oil.

3. Sprinkle onion powder, garlic, and paprika, and then toss it all so that the seasonings blend into the mixture.

4. Bake for 15 minutes until it starts to brown.

5. Remove the vegetables from oven, and then top with shredded Mexican cheese.

6. Place the avocados around the veggies and crack 3 eggs so that they fill the spaces in between. Bake for approximately 10 minutes. Then add cotija cheese, jalapenos (optional), and Tajin on top of eggs.

Macros (per serving)

Calories: 248

Fat: 18g.

Net Carbs: 6g.

Protein: 12g.

Servings: 3

Baked Honey Mustard Chicken

Ingredients

- ✓ 3 Boneless, skinless chicken breasts cut into halves
- ✓ Dash of sea salt
- ✓ Dash of pepper

- ✓ ½ Cup honey
- ✓ ½ Cup mustard
- ✓ 1 Tsp. dried basil
- ✓ 1 Tsp. paprika
- ✓ ½ Tsp. dried parsley

Directions

1. Preheat oven to 350 degrees.

2. Season chicken with sea salt and pepper. Place onto a lightly oiled baking dish.

3. In a bowl, mix together honey, mustard, basil, paprika, and parsley. Pour half of this newly created mixture onto the chicken, and brush to coat.

4. Bake chicken at 350 degrees for 30 minutes. Turn over chicken breasts, and coat with the rest of the honey mix. Bake for 15 more minutes. Allow chicken to cool for at least 10 minutes before serving.

Macros (per serving)

Calories: 232

Fat: 3.7 g.

Net Carbs: 24.8g.

Protein: 25.6g.

Servings: 6

Baked Tilapia

Ingredients

- ✓ 4 Tilapia fillets, 4 ounces each
- ✓ 2 Tsp. butter
- ✓ ¼ Tsp. Old Bay Seasoning
- ✓ ½ Tsp. garlic salt
- ✓ 1 Sliced lemon
- ✓ 16 Oz. package of frozen cauliflower with broccoli and red peppers
- ✓ Dash of sea salt
- ✓ Dash of pepper

Directions

1. Preheat oven to 375 degrees. Lightly oil a baking dish.

2. Place tilapia fillets into the baking dish, and dot them with butter. Then season with Old Bay and garlic salt. Top each fillet with a slice of lemon.

3. Arrange frozen vegetables around the fish evenly, and season with a dash of sea salt and pepper.

4. Cover the baking dish, and bake at 375 degrees for 30 minutes. Vegetables should be tender, and fish should easily flake.

Macros (per serving)

Calories: 172

Fat: 3.6g.

Net Carbs: 7.3g.

Protein: 24.8g.

Servings: 4

Black Bean Chili

Ingredients

- ✓ 1 Tbsp. vegetable oil
- ✓ 1 Diced onion
- ✓ 2 Minced cloves of garlic
- ✓ 1 Lb. ground turkey
- ✓ 3 Cans of undrained black beans (15 ounces each)
- ✓ 1 Can of crushed tomatoes (14 ounces)
- ✓ 1 ½ Tbsp. chili powder
- ✓ 1 Tbsp. dried oregano
- ✓ 1 Tbsp. dried basil leaves
- ✓ 1 Tbsp. red wine vinegar

Directions

1. Heat olive oil in a large pot on medium. Cook onion and garlic until the onion becomes translucent.

2. Add turkey, and cook until meat is brown. Mix in beans, tomatoes, chili powder, oregano, basil, and vinegar. Reduce to low, and simmer for at least one hour.

Macros (per serving)

Calories: 366

Fat: 9.2g.

Net Carbs: 44.1g.

Protein: 29.6g.

Servings: 8

Black Beans and Rice

Ingredients

- ✓ 1 Tsp. olive oil
- ✓ 1 Chopped onion
- ✓ 2 Minced cloves of garlic
- ✓ ¾ Cup brown rice, uncooked
- ✓ ½ Cup vegetable broth (low fat and low sodium)
- ✓ 1 Tsp. ground cumin

- ✓ ¼ Tsp. cayenne pepper
- ✓ 3 ½ Cups canned black beans, drained

Directions

1. Heat oil in a pot on medium. Add onion and garlic. Sauté for approximately 4 minutes.

2. Add rice, and sauté for 2 minutes. Then add vegetable broth, and bring to a boil. Reduce heat, and simmer for 20 minutes.

3. Add all spices and beans. Heat thoroughly.

Macros (per serving)

Calories: 140

Fat: 0.9g.

Net Carbs: 27.1g.

Protein: 6.3g.

Servings: 4

Braised Balsamic Chicken

Ingredients

- ✓ 3 Skinless and boneless chicken breasts cut in half
- ✓ 1 Tsp. garlic salt

- ✓ Dash of sea salt
- ✓ Dash of pepper
- ✓ 2 Tbsp. olive oil
- ✓ 1 Sliced onion
- ✓ 14 Oz. can of diced tomatoes
- ✓ ½ Cup balsamic vinegar
- ✓ 1 Tsp. dried basil
- ✓ 1 Tsp. dried oregano
- ✓ 1 Tsp. dried rosemary
- ✓ ½ Tsp. dried thyme

Directions

1. Rub garlic salt and pepper onto chicken breasts.

2. Heat olive oil in a skillet on medium, and then cook the chicken breasts until they are brown. This takes approximately 4 minutes per side. Then add onion and cook for another 4 minutes.

3. Add tomatoes and vinegar onto the chicken, followed by basil, oregano, rosemary, and thyme. Simmer for 15 minutes or until the chicken is fully cooked.

Macros (per serving)

Calories: 196

Fat: 7 g.

Net Carbs: 7.6g.

Protein: 23.8g.

Servings: 6

Carrot Cake Oatmeal

Ingredients

- ✓ 2/3 Cup fresh pineapple, chopped
- ✓ ½ Cup of sliced carrots
- ✓ 1 Tsp. water
- ✓ 2/3 Cup almond milk
- ✓ ½ Cup old-fashioned oats
- ✓ ½ Tsp. ground cinnamon
- ✓ ½ Tsp ground ginger
- ✓ 1 Tbsp. walnuts, chopped

Directions

1. Mix together pineapple, carrot, and water in a microwave-safe bowl. Cook in microwave for 1 to 2 minutes. The carrots will be partially softened.

2. In another bowl, mix together milk, oats, cinnamon, and ginger into the bowl. Cook in microwave for 1 minute. Then cook in 30 second intervals, stirring oats in between until all oats are tender. Top with walnuts.

Macros (per serving)

Calories: 305

Fat: 9.4g.

Net Carbs: 50.1g.

Protein: 7.9g.

Servings: 2

Chorizo-Spiced Chopped Veggie Salad

Ingredients

- ✓ 1 Head of cauliflower, chopped and removed from stem
- ✓ 2 Chopped cucumbers, seeded
- ✓ 8 Oz. pack of baby carrots, chopped
- ✓ 8 Oz. chopped radish
- ✓ 8 Oz. pack of mushrooms, chopped
- ✓ 4 Oz. chopped cilantro
- ✓ 4 Kale leaves, chopped
- ✓ 1 Large poblano pepper, chopped
- ✓ ½ Cup lime juice
- ✓ ½ Cup white vinegar
- ✓ 2 Tbsp. ground paprika
- ✓ 1 Tbsp. olive oil

- ✓ 1 Tbsp. minced garlic
- ✓ 1 Tbsp. fresh oregano, minced
- ✓ 1 Tbsp. ground cumin
- ✓ 1 Tsp. chili powder
- ✓ ½ Tsp. ground cloves
- ✓ ½ Tsp. ground coriander
- ✓ Dash of sea salt
- ✓ Dash of pepper

Directions

1. Mix together cauliflower, cucumbers, carrots, radishes, mushrooms, cilantro, kale, and poblano pepper in a large bowl with a sealable lid.

2. In a separate bowl, whisk lime juice, vinegar, paprika, olive oil, garlic, oregano, cumin, chili powder, cloves, coriander, salt, and pepper. Make sure that no lumps remain.

3. Pour this mixture over the cauliflower mix in sealable container. Shake until well blended.

Macros (per serving)

Calories: 91

Fat: 2.7g.

Net Carbs: 15.9g.

Protein: 4.5g.

Servings: 8

Creamy Fettuccine with Brussels Sprouts and Mushrooms

Ingredients

- ✓ 4 Cups Brussels sprouts, sliced
- ✓ 12 Oz. fettuccine, whole-wheat
- ✓ 1 Tbsp. extra-virgin olive oil
- ✓ 4 Cups mixed mushrooms, sliced.
- ✓ 1 Tbsp. minced garlic
- ✓ 2 Tbsp. sherry vinegar
- ✓ 2 Cups low-fat milk
- ✓ 2 Tbsp. flour, all-purpose
- ✓ ½ Tsp. salt
- ✓ ½ Tsp. ground pepper
- ✓ 1 Cup Asiago cheese, finely shredded

Directions

1. Boil pasta in a large pot for 10 minutes. Drain away water, and return pasta to pot.

2. While pasta is boiling, use a large skillet to heat the oil on medium. Add in mushrooms and sprouts. Cook for 10 minutes, stirring occasionally. Add garlic, and continue cooking for 1 additional minute. Add in sherry, making sure to scrap up the brown bits. Bring it to a boil until the sherry evaporates. It takes about 10 seconds.

3. Whisk milk and flour on a bowl to the side. Then add mixture to skillet, sprinkling in salt and pepper. Cook approximately 2 minutes, or until the sauce thickens. Mix in Asiago until it fully melts.

4. Add sauce to pasta.

Macros (per serving)

Calories: 384

Fat: 10g.

Carbs: 56g.

Protein: 18g

Total Servings: 6

Curried Cauliflower Steaks with Red Rice
Ingredients

- ✓ 2 Heads of cauliflower
- ✓ 1 Cup red or brown rice
- ✓ 1/3 Cup extra-virgin olive oil
- ✓ 1 Tbsp. lemon juice
- ✓ 2 Tsp. curry powder
- ✓ ½ Tsp. kosher salt

✓ 2 Tbsp. fresh cilantro, chopped

Directions

1. Preheat oven to 450 degrees. Line a large baking sheet with tin foil.

2. Follow directions to prepare rice.

3. Whisk together oil, curry powder, and salt in a bowl.

4. Prepare cauliflower, making sure to keep stems intact. Place stem-side down on a cutting board, and cut into thick slices to create "steaks." Get 4 steaks. Then slice the remaining cauliflower into smaller slices to get 4 cups.

5. Place steaks and florets onto a baking sheet. Brush both sides of the steaks with the curry mixture.

6. Place steaks in oven, turning after 15 minutes. Finish baking until steaks are tender and brown.

7. Divide rice evenly onto 4 plates, and top each plate with a cauliflower steak. Sprinkle with cilantro.

Note: You can refrigerate cauliflower for up to 3 days so you can prepare it ahead of time if needed.

Macros (per serving)

Calories: 410

Fat: 21g.

Carbs: 49g.

Protein: 10g

Total Servings: 4

Garlic Chicken with Orzo Noodles

Ingredients

- ✓ 1 Cup uncooked orzo pasta
- ✓ 2 Tbsp. olive oil
- ✓ 2 Cloves of garlic
- ✓ ¼ Tsp. crushed red pepper
- ✓ 1 Skinless and boneless chicken breast, cut into bite-sized pieces
- ✓ Dash of sea salt
- ✓ 1 Tbsp. chopped parsley
- ✓ 2 Cups fresh spinach
- ✓ Parmesan cheese to taste (for topping)

Directions

1. Bring a large pot of lightly salted water to a boil. Add in the pasta, and cook for approximately 10 minutes, or until the pasta is al dente. Drain.

2. Heat olive oil in a skillet on medium. Cook garlic and red pepper for 1 minute. Add chicken and cook for 5 minutes, seasoning with sea salt. Add parsley and cooked orzo. Finally, place spinach into the skillet and cook for 5 more minutes.

3. Top with Parmesan cheese.

Macros (per serving)

Calories: 351

Fat: 10.6 g.

Net Carbs: 40.4g.

Protein: 22.3g.

Servings: 2

Ginger Mahi Mahi

Ingredients

- ✓ 3 Tbsp. honey
- ✓ 3 Tbsp. soy sauce
- ✓ 3 Tbsp. balsamic vinegar
- ✓ 1 Tsp. fresh ginger root
- ✓ 1 Clove garlic, crushed
- ✓ 2 Tsp. olive oil
- ✓ 1 Mahi Mahi fillets, 6 ounces each
- ✓ Dash of sea salt
- ✓ Dash of pepper

✓ 1 Tbsp. vegetable oil

Directions

1. Mix together honey, soy sauce, balsamic vinegar, ginger, garlic, and olive oil in a small glass dish.

2. Season fillets with salt and pepper before placing them into the dish with the honey mix. Cover dish and place in the refrigerator for 20 minutes.

3. Heat vegetable oil in a skillet on medium, and then place fish into the skillet. Save the marinade for later. Cook fish for 4 minutes on each side, turning only one time. Remove from skillet and place onto a platter.

4. Pour the saved marinade into the skillet until it reduces to a glaze. Spoon this glaze over fish and serve immediately.

Macros (per serving)

Calories: 259

Fat: 7 g.

Net Carbs: 16g.

Protein: 32.4g.

Servings: 4

Heart-Healthy Chicken Stew

Ingredients

- ✓ 2 Tbsp. olive oil
- ✓ 2 Skinless, boneless chicken breasts cut into cubes
- ✓ 2 Sweet potatoes cut into cubes
- ✓ ½ Chopped red onion
- ✓ 1 Cubed small eggplant
- ✓ 2 Minced cloves of garlic
- ✓ 1 Tbsp. minced fresh ginger root
- ✓ 2 Tsp. ground turmeric
- ✓ ½ Cup chicken broth, low sodium

Directions

1. In a large skillet, heat olive oil on medium. Add in chicken, and cook until it's brown in the center. This will take approximately 5 minutes.

2. Add sweet potatoes and onion to the skillet. Cook for approximately 3 minutes, or until onion is translucent.

3. Add eggplant, garlic, ginger, and turmeric to the skillet. Continue cooking for 1 more minute until it becomes fragrant. Then pour in broth and simmer, cooking until the stew thickens. This will take approximately 20 minutes.

Macros (per serving)

Calories: 183

Fat: 5.5g.

Net Carbs: 24.1g.

Protein: 9.9g.

Servings: 4

Lemon-Garlic Shrimp over Orzo with Zucchini

Ingredients

- ✓ 1 ½ Lbs. large shrimp in shells, either fresh or frozen
- ✓ 2 Lemons
- ✓ ¾ Cup orzo pasta, dried
- ✓ 2 Tbsp. olive oil
- ✓ 1 Tbsp. butter, unsalted
- ✓ 3 Cloves minced garlic
- ✓ 1/8 Tsp. red pepper, crushed
- ✓ 2 Cups zucchini, sliced
- ✓ ¼ Cup shallots, thinly sliced
- ✓ ¼ Tsp. black pepper
- ✓ 2 Tbsp. water
- ✓ 1 Tsp. fresh rosemary, snipped
- ✓ 2 Tbsp. fresh dill weed, snipped

Directions

1. Peel shrimp. You can leave tails intact if you want. Thoroughly rinse shrimp, and use a paper towel to pat them dry.

2. Remove zest from 1 lemon using a vegetable peeler, cutting into thin slivers. Squeeze ¼ cup of juice from lemons. You should have half a lemon left. Place it to the side.

3. Prepare orzo following the instructions on the package. Leave out any salt and fat.

4. Heat up oil and butter in a nonstick skillet on medium-high. Add in shrimp, 2 cloves of garlic, ¼ Tsp. salt, and crushed red pepper.

5. Cook shrimp for approximately 2 minutes or until they are opaque. Mix in lemon juice.

6. Remove from heat, and cover so that it stays warm.

7. Heat remaining oil in the skillet. Add zucchini, shallots, pepper, the remaining garlic clove, and ¼ tsp. salt. Cook for 3 minutes until the zucchini is light brown.

8. Add in rosemary, water, and the rest of the lemon juice. Stir so that you scrape up the crusty bits. Mix in the cooked orzo.

9. Stir in shrimp mix, and sprinkle with dill and slivers of lemon. Finally, squeeze the juice from the remaining half lemon over the mixture.

Macros (per serving)

Calories: 355

Fat: 11g.

Carbs: 30g.

Protein: 35g

Total Servings: 4

Mediterranean Chicken with Orzo Salad

Ingredients

- ✓ 2 Skinless, boneless chicken breasts cut into halves
- ✓ 3 Tbsp. extra-virgin olive oil
- ✓ 1 Tsp. lemon zest
- ✓ ½ Tsp. salt
- ✓ ½ Tsp. pepper
- ✓ ¾ Cup whole-wheat orzo
- ✓ 2 Cups baby spinach, thinly sliced
- ✓ 1 Cup cucumber, chopped
- ✓ 1 Cup tomato, chopped
- ✓ ¼ Cup red onion, chopped
- ✓ ¼ Cup feta cheese, crumbled

- ✓ 2 Tbsp. Kalamata onions, chopped
- ✓ 2 Tbsp. lemon juice
- ✓ 1 Clove garlic, grated
- ✓ 2 Tsp. fresh oregano, chopped

Directions

1. Preheat over at 425 degrees

2. Brush 1 Tbsp. olive oil over chicken and then sprinkle with lemon zest and ¼ Tsp. salt and pepper. Place chicken into a baking dish.

3. Bake 30 minutes or until thermometer registers at 165 degrees inside of the chicken.

4. While chicken is baking in the oven, bring a saucepan of water to a boil. Add orzo, and then cook for approximately 8 minutes. Add spinach and cook for 1 additional minute. Drain and then rinse with cold water.

5. Transfer spinach and orzo to a large bowl. Add cucumber, tomato, onion, feta, and olives. Mix together.

6. In a small bowl, whisk remaining olive oil, lemon juice oregano, salt, and pepper. Then mix all just 1 Tbsp. of the dressing mix into the orzo mixture. Drizzle remaining 1 Tbsp. over chicken and serve with the salad.

Macros (per serving)

Calories: 400

Fat: 7g.

Carbs: 28g.

Protein: 32g

Total Servings: 4

Old Fashioned Potato Salad

Ingredients

- ✓ 5 Potatoes
- ✓ 3 Eggs
- ✓ 1 Cup chopped celery
- ✓ ½ Cup chopped onion
- ✓ ½ Cup pickle relish
- ✓ ¼ Tsp. garlic salt
- ✓ ¼ Tsp. celery salt
- ✓ 1 Tbsp. mustard
- ✓ Dash of pepper
- ✓ ¼ Cup mayonnaise

Directions

1. Bring a large pot of lightly salted water to a boil. Add in potatoes, and boil until they are tender. This will take approximately 15 minutes. Drain the potatoes before peeling and chopping them.

2. Place eggs into a saucepan, and then cover them with cold water. Bring water to a boil. Remove from heat and cover. Allow the eggs to stand in the cold water for 12 minutes. Remove, peel, and chop eggs into cubes.

3. Mix together potatoes, eggs, celery, onion, relish, garlic salt, celery salt, mustard, pepper, and mayonnaise in a large bowl. Refrigerate and serve cold.

Macros (per serving)

Calories: 206

Fat: 7.6g.

Net Carbs: 30.5g.

Protein: 5.5g.

Servings: 6

Peanut-Butter Cinnamon Toast

Ingredients

- ✓ 1 Slice toasted bread, whole-wheat
- ✓ 1 Tbsp. peanut butter
- ✓ 1 Banana
- ✓ Cinnamon (to taste)

Directions

1. Spread peanut butter onto toast. Top it with banana slices. Then sprinkle with cinnamon to taste.

Macros (per serving)

Calories: 266

Fat: 9g.

Carbs: 38g.

Protein: 8g

Total Servings: 1

Penne Pasta with Spinach and Bacon

Ingredients

- ✓ 1 Package of penne pasta (12 ounces)
- ✓ 2 Tbsp. olive oil
- ✓ 6 Slices of bacon, chopped
- ✓ 2 Tbsp. garlic, minced
- ✓ 1 Can of diced tomatoes (14 ounces)
- ✓ 1 Bunch of fresh spinach, torn into bite-sized pieces

Directions

1. Bring a large pot of lightly salted water to a boil, and then add in the penne pasta. Cook for approximately 10 minutes or until the pasta is tender.

2. Heat up 1 Tbsp. olive oil in a skillet on medium. Then place bacon in the skillet, and cook until crisp. Add in the garlic, and cook for another minute. Stir in tomatoes, and continue cooking until mixture is thoroughly heated.

3. Place spinach into a colander, and drain pasta over it so that it wilts. Transfer it to a large serving bowl, and then toss with remaining olive oil and bacon mixture.

Macros (per serving)

Calories: 517

Fat: 14.8g.

Net Carbs: 73.8g.

Protein: 21g.

Servings: 4

Quinoa and Black Beans

Ingredients

- ✓ 1 Tsp. olive oil
- ✓ 1 Chopped onion
- ✓ 3 Cloves of garlic, chopped
- ✓ ¾ Cup quinoa
- ✓ 1 ½ Cups vegetable broth
- ✓ 1 Tsp. ground cumin
- ✓ ¼ Tsp. cayenne pepper

- ✓ Dash of sea salt
- ✓ Dash of pepper
- ✓ 1 Cup frozen corn
- ✓ 2-15 Oz. cans of black beans, rinsed and drained
- ✓ ½ Cup fresh cilantro, chopped

Directions

1. Heat olive oil in a saucepan on medium. Cook onion and garlic for approximately 10 minutes until it is lightly browned.

2. Mix in quinoa with the onions and garlic. Cover with vegetable broth, and then season with cumin, cayenne pepper, salt, and pepper.

3. Bring mix to a boil, and then reduce heat. Simmer until quinoa is tender and broth is absorbed, which takes about 20 minutes.

4. Mix frozen corn into a saucepan, and continue to simmer until it has been thoroughly heated.

Macros (per serving)

Calories: 153

Fat: 1.7g.

Net Carbs: 27.8g.

Protein: 7.7g.

Servings: 6

Quinoa Meatless Balls

Ingredients

- ✓ 2 ½ Cup quinoa, cooked
- ✓ 4 Eggs
- ✓ ½ Tsp. salt
- ✓ 1/3 Cup chives
- ✓ 1 Onion
- ✓ 1/3 Cup Parmesan cheese, grated
- ✓ 3 Cloves garlic
- ✓ 1 ¾ Cup bread crumbs, whole grain
- ✓ 1 Tbsp. extra virgin olive oil

Directions

1. Combine ingredients in a large bowl. Mix thoroughly.

2. Using your hands, create meatballs from the mixture.

3. Coat a skillet with olive oil.

4. Cook meatballs in the skillet for approximately 10 minutes, until brown.

Macros (per serving)

Calories: 291

Fat: 10g.

Carbs: 139g.

Protein: 13g

Total Servings: 12

Roasted New Potatoes

Ingredients

- ✓ 3 Lbs. new potatoes, cut into halves
- ✓ ¼ Cup olive oil
- ✓ Dash of sea salt
- ✓ Dash of pepper

Directions

1. Move oven rack to the lowest position. Preheat oven to 450 degrees. Toss together potatoes with oil, sea salt, and pepper. Arrange the coated potatoes with the cut side down onto a large cookie sheet.

2. Roast potatoes at 450 degrees for approximately 30 minutes. They will be tender and golden brown.

Macros (per serving)

Calories: 179

Fat: 7g.

Net Carbs: 27.1g.

Protein: 3.2g.

Servings: 6

Salsa Chicken Burrito Filling

Ingredients

- ✓ 1 Skinless and boneless chicken breast, cut in half
- ✓ 1 Can of tomato sauce (4 ounces)
- ✓ ¼ Cup salsa
- ✓ 1 Package of taco seasoning
- ✓ 1 Tsp. ground cumin
- ✓ 2 Cloves of minced garlic
- ✓ 1 Tsp. chili powder
- ✓ Hot sauce (to taste)

Directions

1. Place chicken breasts and tomato sauce in a medium sized saucepan on medium heat. Bring the sauce to a boil, and then add salsa, seasoning, cumin, garlic, and chili powder. Let this mixture simmer for 15 minutes.

2. Use a fork to pull apart the chicken, forming thin strings. Then keep cooking the pulled chicken meat and sauce for 10 more minutes. Add hot sauce to taste.

Macros (per serving)

Calories: 107

Fat: 1.5g.

Net Carbs: 9.6g.

Protein: 12.3g.

Servings: 2

Sausage Egg Muffins

Ingredients

- ✓ ½ Lb. pork sausage, ground
- ✓ 12 Beaten eggs
- ✓ 2 Oz. Chopped chili peppers, green
- ✓ 1 Chopped onion
- ✓ 1 tsp. garlic powder
- ✓ Dash of salt
- ✓ Dash of black pepper

Directions

1. Preheat oven to 350 degrees. Lightly oil a set of 12 muffin cups.

2. Cook sausage in a skillet until it is brown. Drain it and place to the side.

3. Mix together eggs, chilis, onion, garlic powder, salt, pepper, and sausage in a bowl.

4. Add this new mixture evenly to the muffin cups.

5. Bake at 350 degrees for 15 minutes or until eggs are done.

Macros (per serving)

Calories: 155

Fat: 13g.

Net Carbs: 2g.

Protein: 9g.

Servings: 12

Smoked Salmon Fried Rice

Ingredients

- ✓ 6 Cups water
- ✓ 2 Cups uncooked brown rice, long grain
- ✓ 3 Tbsp. olive oil
- ✓ 2 Eggs
- ✓ ½ Onion, chopped
- ✓ 1 Green onion, chopped
- ✓ 4 Oz. smoked salmon
- ✓ ½ Cup of frozen peas

- ✓ Dash of salt
- ✓ Dash of pepper

Directions

1. Add water to a saucepan. Then add rice, and bring water to a boil. Reduce heat to low and cover. Allow rice to simmer for approximately 20 minutes.

2. While rice simmers, add 2 Tbsp. olive oil to a large skillet and heat on medium. Mix in eggs, and cook until they are scrambled. Remove eggs and place to the side.

3. Use the same skillet. Add 1 Tbsp. olive oil, and heat on medium. Add onion and green onion, cooking for about 5 minutes or until it's transparent. Mix in salmon, rice, peas, and eggs until it's all well-blended. Continue cooking and stirring rice mixture until it has been thoroughly heated. Use salt and pepper to season.

Macros (per serving)

Calories: 458

Fat: 10g.

Net Carbs: 76.8g.

Protein: 12.9g.

Servings: 4

Spicy Avocado

Ingredients

- ✓ 1 Cup of ripe, halved avocado
- ✓ ½ Juiced lemon
- ✓ 2 Tbsp. hot sauce
- ✓ Dash of sea salt

Directions

1. Slice the avocado in half a few times; spin and slice a few more times perpendicular to the first slices. You should end up with several cubes that are still attached to the peel.

2. Drizzle the lemon juice and hot sauce onto the avocado. Eat with a fork.

Macros (per serving)

Calories: 124

Fat: 10.8g.

Net Carbs: 9.5g.

Protein: 1.9g.

Servings: 1

Spicy Black-Eyed Peas

Ingredients

- ✓ 6 Cups water
- ✓ 1 Cube of chicken bouillon
- ✓ 1 Lb. black-eyes peas, dry and rinsed
- ✓ 1 Diced onion
- ✓ 2 Diced cloves of garlic
- ✓ 1 Diced red bell pepper
- ✓ 1 Minced jalapeno
- ✓ 8 Oz. diced ham
- ✓ 4 Chopped slices of bacon
- ✓ ½ Tsp. cayenne pepper
- ✓ 1 ½ Tsp. cumin
- ✓ Dash of sea salt
- ✓ Dash of pepper

Directions

1. Pour water into a slow cooker, and then add bouillon cube. Stir until the cube dissolves.

2. Add black-eyed peas, onion, garlic, bell pepper, jalapeno pepper, ham, bacon, cayenne pepper, cumin, salt, and pepper. Stir together to blend, and then cover the cooker. Cook for approximately 6 hours until the beans are tender.

Macros (per serving)

Calories: 199

Fat: 2.9g.

Net Carbs: 30.2g.

Protein: 14.1g.

Servings: 8

Split Pea Soup

Ingredients

- ✓ 2 ¼ Cup dried split peas
- ✓ 2 Quarts cold water
- ✓ 1 ½ Lb. ham bone
- ✓ 2 Sliced onions
- ✓ ½ Tsp. sea salt
- ✓ ½ Tsp pepper
- ✓ Pinch of dried marjoram
- ✓ 3 Stalks of celery, chopped
- ✓ 3 Carrots, chopped
- ✓ 1 Diced potato

Directions

PREPARATION: Using a large pot, cover the peas with 2 quarts of cold water, and allow it to soak overnight. You can also simmer the peas for 2 minutes, and then allow them to soak for 1 hour.

1. Add ham bone, onion, salt, pepper, and marjoram. Cover pot, and bring mixture to a boil. Simmer for 90 minutes, stirring occasionally.

2. Remove bone, and cut away the meat. Dice and return it to the soup. Add celery, carrots, and potatoes. Slowly cook the soup for 30 minutes uncovered. Vegetables will be tender when the soup is finished.

<u>**Macros (per serving)**</u>

Calories: 310

Fat: 1g.

Net Carbs: 57.9g.

Protein: 19.7g.

Servings: 6

Stuffed Sweet Potato with Hummus Dressing

<u>**Ingredients**</u>

- ✓ 1 Sweet potato, scrubbed
- ✓ ¾ Cup kale, chopped
- ✓ 1 Cup canned black beans, rinsed

✓ ¼ Cup hummus

✓ 2 Tbsp. water

Directions

1. Poke small holes into the sweet potato using a fork. Microwave on high until it's fully cooked.

2. Wash kale, and allow a small amount of water to cling to leaves. Place into a saucepan, cover, and cook on medium. Stir 2 times before adding beans and add 1 Tbsp. water if pot is dry. Cook until mixture is steaming hot.

3. Cut open the sweet potato, and top with the kale mixture. Combine hummus and 2 Tbsp water in a separate dish. Add additional water if needed.

4. Drizzle hummus dressing over sweet potatoes.

Macros (per serving)
Calories: 472
Fat: 7g.
Carbs: 85g.
Protein: 21g
Total Servings: 1

Sweet Potato Breakfast Bake
Ingredients

- ✓ 1 Tbsp. olive oil
- ✓ 1 Diced sweet potato
- ✓ 1 Lb. sausage
- ✓ ½ Cup chopped onion
- ✓ ½ Diced red bell pepper
- ✓ 1 Cup mushroom, sliced
- ✓ 1 Cup kale leaves, torn
- ✓ Dash of salt
- ✓ Dash of black pepper
- ✓ 5 Eggs
- ✓ 1/3 Cup water
- ✓ 1 Tsp. thyme, dried
- ✓ 1 Green onion, diced

Directions

1. Preheat oven to 400 degrees.

2. In a skillet, heat olive oil before adding sweet potato. Cook covered for approximately 8 minutes, stirring occasionally. Transfer sweet potato into a large bowl.

3. Using the same skillet, cook the sausage on medium until it is brown and crumbled, approximately 4-5 minutes. Add sausage to the bowl with the sweet potato.

4. Using the same skillet, cook onion and bell pepper for approximately 3 minutes, and then season it with salt and pepper. Add mushrooms and kale. Cook for approximately 3 minutes. Transfer it to the bowl with sausage and sweet potato.

5. In a bowl, whisk together eggs, water, thyme, salt, and pepper. Mix in sausage mixture. Pour this new mix into a baking dish.

6. Bake at 400 degrees for approximately 20-25 minutes, until the sweet potato starts to brown. Garnish it with the onion.

Macros (per serving)

Calories: 489

Fat: 34g.

Net Carbs: 20g.

Protein: 26g.

Servings: 4

Tuna Salad Sandwich

Ingredients

- ✓ 1 Can white tuna, unsalted and packed in water
- ✓ ¼ Cup celery, diced
- ✓ ½ Tsp. lemon juice
- ✓ ¼ Cup low-calorie mayonnaise
- ✓ 2 Slices bread, whole-wheat

Directions

1. Fluff tuna with a fork in a small bowl, and then add the rest of the ingredients. Mix thoroughly.

2. Spread the mixture evenly over one slice of bread so that you create two sandwiches.

Note: You will have half of the mixture left over. You can make another sandwich with it later. It can be stored in the refrigerator for up to one day.

Macros (per serving)

Calories: 240

Fat: 3g.

Carbs: 24g.

Protein: 19g

Total Servings: 2 (read note)

Turkey Veggie Meatload Cups

Ingredients

- ✓ 2 Cups zucchini, chopped
- ✓ 1 ½ Cup onions, chopped
- ✓ 1 Red bell pepper, chopped
- ✓ 1 Lb. ground turkey

- ✓ ½ Cup uncooked couscous
- ✓ 1 Egg
- ✓ 2 Tbsp. Worcestershire sauce
- ✓ 1 Tbsp. Dijon mustard
- ✓ ½ Cup barbeque sauce

Directions

1. Preheat oven to 400 degrees. Lightly oil or spray 20 muffin cups.

2. Mix together zucchini, onions, and red bell pepper using a food processor. They should be finely chopped but not liquefied. Place this mixture into a bowl, and mix in the ground turkey, couscous, egg, Worcestershire sauce, and Dijon mustard until it has been thoroughly combined.

3. Fill oiled muffin cups with this newly created mixture. They should be about ¾ of the way full. Top each with approximately 1 Tsp. of barbeque sauce.

4. Bake at 400 degrees for approximately 25 minutes. The internal temperature of each muffin should be 160 degrees. Let cups stand for 5 minutes before serving.

Macros (per serving)

Calories: 119

Fat: 1g.

Net Carbs: 13.6g.

Protein: 13.2g.

Servings: 10

Ultimate Breakfast Roll Ups

Ingredients

- ✓ 10 Large eggs
- ✓ Dash of sea salt
- ✓ Dash of ground black pepper
- ✓ 1 ½ Cups cheddar cheese, shredded
- ✓ 5 Slices cooked bacon
- ✓ 5 Cooked breakfast sausage patties
- ✓ Nonstick cooking spray

Directions

1. Whisk 2 eggs in a bowl, and then cook them in a skillet on medium. You should spray the skillet with nonstick spray before placing eggs into it. Season these eggs with sea salt and pepper. Cover skillet while eggs thoroughly cook.

2. Sprinkle 1/3 cup of cheese on the eggs. Lay down one strip of bacon, and then top that with sausage patty. You will then need to carefully fold the egg until it looks like a breakfast burrito.

3. Repeat this until you have 5 breakfast rolls.

Macros (per serving)

Calories: 412

Fat: 31g.

Net Carbs: 2g.

Protein: 28g.

Servings: 5

Veggie-Hummus Sandwich

Ingredients

- ✓ 2 slices of bread, whole-grain
- ✓ ¼ Avocado, mashed
- ✓ 3 Tbsp. Hummus
- ✓ ½ Cup salad greens
- ✓ ¼ Medium bell pepper, red and sliced
- ✓ ¼ Cup sliced cucumber
- ✓ ¼ Cup shredded carrot

Directions

1. Spread hummus on one side of bread and avocado on the other side.

2. Fill the sandwich with the remainder of ingredients.

3. Slice in half.

Note: You can make this 4 hours ahead of time if you store it in the refrigerator.

Macros (per serving)

Calories: 325

Fat: 14g.

Carbs: 40g.

Protein: 13g

Total Servings: 1

White Bean and Avocado Salad

Ingredients

- ✓ 2 Cups salad greens, mixed and fresh
- ✓ ¾ Cup fresh vegetables chopped, your choice.
- ✓ 1/3 Cup canned white beans
- ✓ 1/2 Avocado, diced
- ✓ 2 Tbsp. all-purpose vinaigrette

Directions

1. Toss everything together in a bowl to create your delicious salad.

Macros (per serving)

Calories: 230

Fat: 16g.

Carbs: 15g.

Protein: 9g

Total Servings: 1

White Bean Chicken Chili

Ingredients

- ✓ 2 Tbsp. olive oil
- ✓ 1 Chopped onion
- ✓ 2 Cloves of minced garlic
- ✓ 1 Can chicken broth (14 ounces)
- ✓ 1 Can Tomatillos (18 ounces) chopped and drained
- ✓ 1 Can diced tomatoes (16 ounces)
- ✓ 1 Can diced green chilis (7 ounces)
- ✓ ½ Tsp. dried oregano
- ✓ ½ Tsp. ground coriander seed
- ✓ ¼ Tsp. ground cumin
- ✓ 2 Ears of fresh corn
- ✓ 1 Lb. chicken, cooked and diced
- ✓ 1 Can white beans (15 ounces)
- ✓ Dash of sea salt

✓ Dash of pepper

Directions

1. Heat oil, and cook onion and garlic in a sauce pan until soft.

2. Add broth, tomatillos, tomatoes, chilies, and spices. Thoroughly mix them together and then bring it to a boil. Simmer for 10 minutes.

3. Add in the corn, chicken, and beans. Simmer for 5 additional minutes. Season with sea salt and pepper.

Macros (per serving)

Calories: 220

Fat: 6.1g.

Net Carbs: 21.2g.

Protein: 20.1g.

Servings: 8

Yogurt with Nuts and Raspberries

Ingredients

✓ 1 Cup Green yogurt, plain and nonfat
✓ ½ Cup raspberries
✓ 5 walnuts, chopped

✓ 1 Tsp. honey

Directions

1. Place raspberries, honey, and walnuts on top of yogurt.

Macros (per serving)

Calories: 250

Fat: 4.5g.

Carbs: 35g.

Protein: 19g

Total Servings: 1

Conversion Tables

U.S. Standard	U.S. St. Ounces	Metric
2 Tbsp.	1 fl. Oz.	30 mL
1/4 Cup	2 fl. Oz.	60 mL
1/2 Cup	4 fl. Oz.	120 mL
1 Cup	8 fl. Oz.	240 mL
1 ½ Cup	12 fl. Oz.	355 mL
2 Cups	16 fl. Oz.	475 mL
4 Cups	32 fl. Oz.	1 L
1 Gallon	128 fl. Oz.	4 L

Oven Temperatures

Fahrenheit (F)	Celsius (C)
250 F	120 C
300 F	150 C
325 F	165 C
350 F	180 C
375 F	190 C
400 F	200 C
425 F	220 C
450 F	230 C

Liquid Volume

Standard U.S.	Metric
1/8 Tsp.	0.5 mL
1/4 Tsp.	1 mL
1/2 Tsp.	2 mL
2/3 Tsp.	4 mL
1 Tsp.	5 mL
1 Tbsp.	15 mL
1/4 Cup	59 mL
1/3 Cup	79 mL
1/2 Cup	118 mL
2/3 Cup	156 mL
3/4 Cup	177 mL
1 Cup	235 mL
2 Cups / 1 Pint	475 mL
3 Cups	700 mL
4 Cups / 1 Quart	1 L
1/2 Gallon	2 L
1 Gallon	4 L

Weight Conversion

U.S. Standard	Metric
1/2 Ounce	15 g
1 Ounce	30 g
2 Ounces	60 g
4 Ounces	115 g
8 Ounces	225 g
12 Ounces	340 g
16 Ounces / 1 Pound	455 g

One Last Thing... Did You Enjoy the Book?

If so, then let me know by leaving a review on Amazon! Reviews are the lifeblood of independent authors. I would appreciate even a few words from you!

If you did not like the book, then please tell me! Email me at lizard.publishing@gmail.com and let me know what you didn't like. Perhaps I can change it. In today's world, a book doesn't have to be stagnant. It should be improved with time and feedback from readers like you. You can impact this book, and I welcome your feedback. Help me make this book better for everyone!